Famous Doctors

A Brief Biography of Medicine

Steve Petty, MD

ISBN: 1494906368
ISBN-13: 9781494906368
Library of Congress Control Number: **XXXXX (If applicable)**
LCCN Imprint Name: **City and State (If applicable**

To Hershel, a great brother and mentor.

About the Author

Steve Petty enjoys music, sports, and travel. He is a primary care physician in San Jose, California. He graduated from UC Irvine Medical School and completed a San Jose (Stanford-affiliated) family practice residency. He is board-certified in both family medicine and sports medicine, and he is an adjunct clinical assistant professor at Stanford Medical School Department of Family Medicine. He plays guitar and sings in the band Petty Therapy. Dr. Petty also writes a quarterly investment column.

Other Books by the Author

The Allergy Epidemic: Understanding and Treating Environmental
Allergies
Affirmations: Guides to Feel Good about Yourself
Petty Therapy Song Book
Poetry: A Young Life in Poems

Music CDs produced and played by the author
It's a Good Life
Live at 9 Lives Club
Love Songs
Take this Monkey off My Back
Silicon Valley Blues
I Want to Sing

All Books and CDs are available on Amazon.com.
Visit Steve Petty's website: amazon.com/author/stevepettymd.

There are in fact two things, science and opinion; the former begets knowledge, the latter ignorance

Hippocrates

We doctors have always been a simple trusting folk. Did we not believe Galen implicitly for 1500 years, and Hippocrates for more than 2000 years?

William Osler

Science has everything to say about what is possible. Science has nothing to say about what is permissible.

Charles Krauthammer

Famous Doctors

Table of Contents

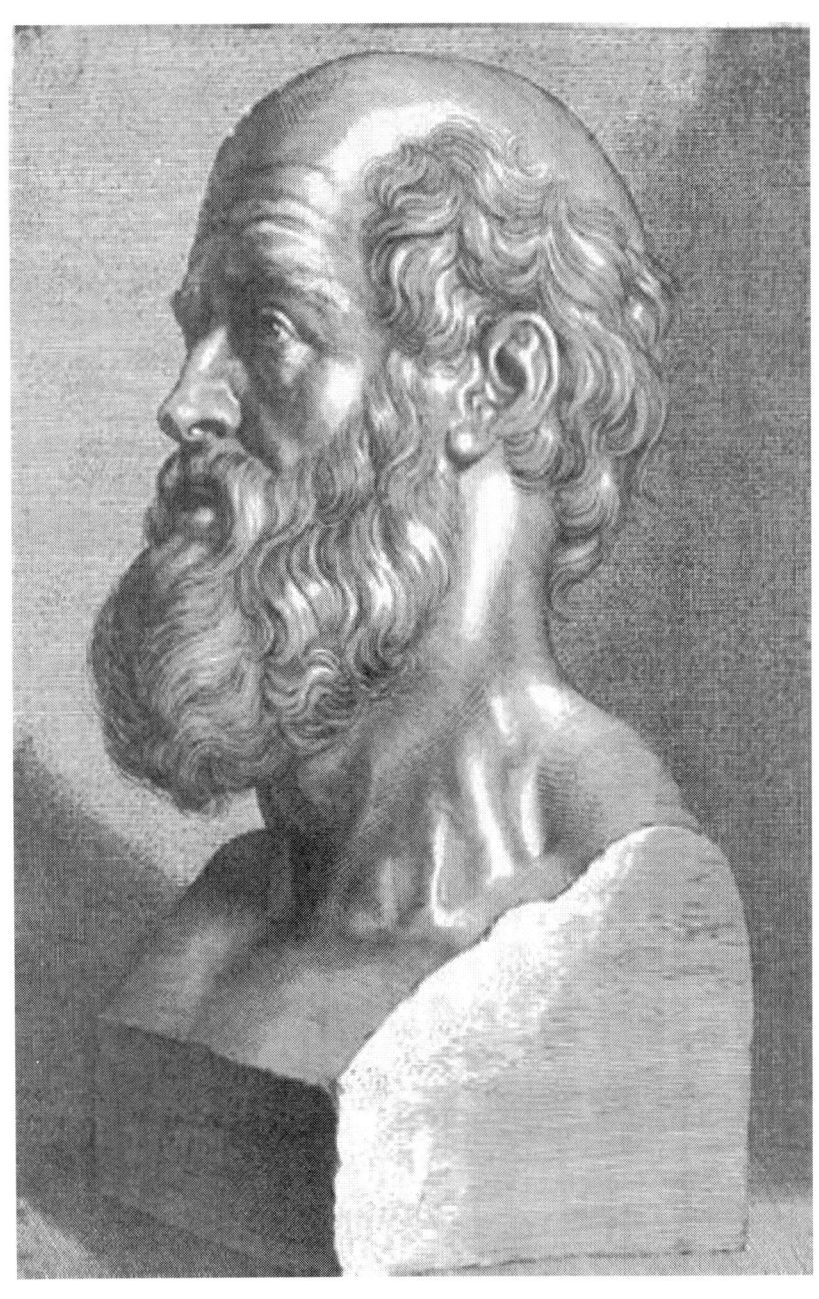

Hippocrates

Hippocrates (*ca.* 460–377 BC)

We know very little about the life of Hippocrates, a short man from the Greek island of Cos, who is known as the father of medicine. He probably learned medicine from his father, as medicine was a hereditary profession in Greece. Now we remember him for his phrase *Primum non nocere* (First, do no harm) and the Hippocratic oath, which historians doubt he actually wrote himself. An enormous work called the *Corpus Hippocraticum* (works of Hippocrates) was arranged by Ptolemy, who commissioned Egyptian scholars to collect all the works of Hippocrates. These scholars obtained some seventy works; however, only twenty are considered actually written by Hippocrates himself.

Hippocrates's book *On Epidemics* emphasized that medical art consisted of three main elements: "the disease, the patient, and the physician." Before and even after this thinking, disease was believed to be of divine providence and cured by divine rite. Hippocrates saw the patient as an individual whose "constitution will react to disease in its own way."

As a physician, his main service to patients was to observe, classify and predict the course of disease. He knew that the course of a disease was affected by the patient's environment and way of life. Further, he recognized that there was nothing sacred about sickness, but certain ailments often followed predictable patterns. He recorded symptoms of specific diseases, and after seeing similar patterns, he could give a prognosis. Giving a patient and family a prognosis would, he said, "help the patient and impress his family." Since many of his pharmaceuticals were ineffective, one of his most significant services was to give an accurate prognosis of a patient's illness.

The Greek philosophical approach to a patient was that a physician assists nature's healing process. To do this, a physician must know the disease, its course, and its possible final outcome. He must taste the patient's urine, sputum, stool, and other body fluids and listen to a patient's lungs. Hippocrates had little knowledge of internal human anatomy because human dissection was not studied in his time period. Anatomy was studied by examining the external human body only. Gross external changes were recognized more easily by Hippocrates, and for this reason, his medicine was more surgical and less medicinal. For example, an abscess or a broken leg with deformity or shoulder dislocation would be considered a treatable condition to him.

In his *Epidemics*, Hippocrates wrote detailed descriptions of diseases and was the first to coin the term epidemic. He believed that disease had a cause-and-effect relationship and was not related to gods. Some diseases were related to bad humors, ill-regulated living, and unsuitable food. Minor ailments were often treated by resting, dieting, and eating light broth. For serious illness, purgatives, emetics, and bleedings were carried out. Bleeding a patient was believed to help balance the disequilibrium of excessive internal humors.

The humoral theory of medicine in Greece in the time of Hippocrates was based on the fundamental concept that nature seeks to maintain a condition of stability—what we today call homeostasis. A physician was to discover a disease's course and support nature in restoring balance to the person. Nature accomplished this cure by driving out the humors.

Hippocrates believed that a pepsis or coction was made by the body to cause *innate heat*, which ripened or cooked the noxious humor into a form that could be expelled as pus, phlegm, diarrhea, gastrointestinal bleeding, nasal discharge, or sputum.

Greek physicians assumed a fever made the phlegm so that it could be expelled. For example, pneumonia or a sinus infection would cause a fever and make a patient bring up phlegm. The body came to what was called a crisis, and at that very moment recovery occurred dramatically—or the patient died. During the crisis, lysis of the illness-causing humors caused them to be expelled, resulting in a cure.

The portion of the *Corpus Hippocraticum* that survives today forms the basis of modern medicine. Hippocrates's work gives an excellent account of diseases and the thought process as the Greeks interpreted disease during the period 300 to 400 BC. During the Dark Ages, also called the Middle Ages, between about AD 700 to 1100, medical intervention was considered "divine intervention." Hippocrates's works were not considered in the medical community again until the Italian Renaissance, from about the fourteenth to sixteenth centuries.

By the fourteen hundreds and fifteen hundreds, anatomy was being studied, which made many of Hippocrates's works obsolete. However, his careful observation and study of the patient and disease gave him the honorary distinction of the *Father of Medicine*. Even today, medical students read the Hippocratic oath when graduating from medical school.

Contemporaries of Hippocrates were Socrates, Plato, and Sophocles. In this Greek period 300-400 BC advances in science, philosophy, mathematics and medicine were to lay a foundation of western culture and learning.

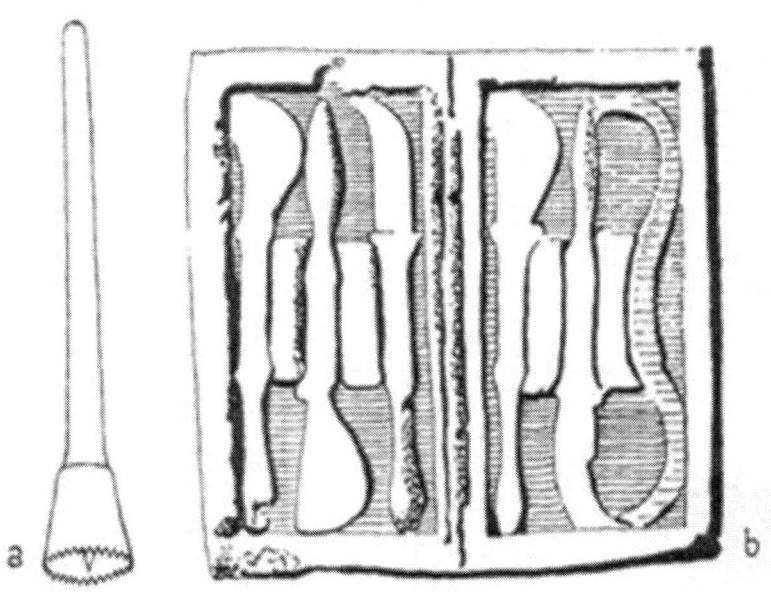

Types of scalpels and instruments used by doctors in the time of Hippocrates.

"The natural healing force within each of us is the greatest force in getting well." Hippocrates

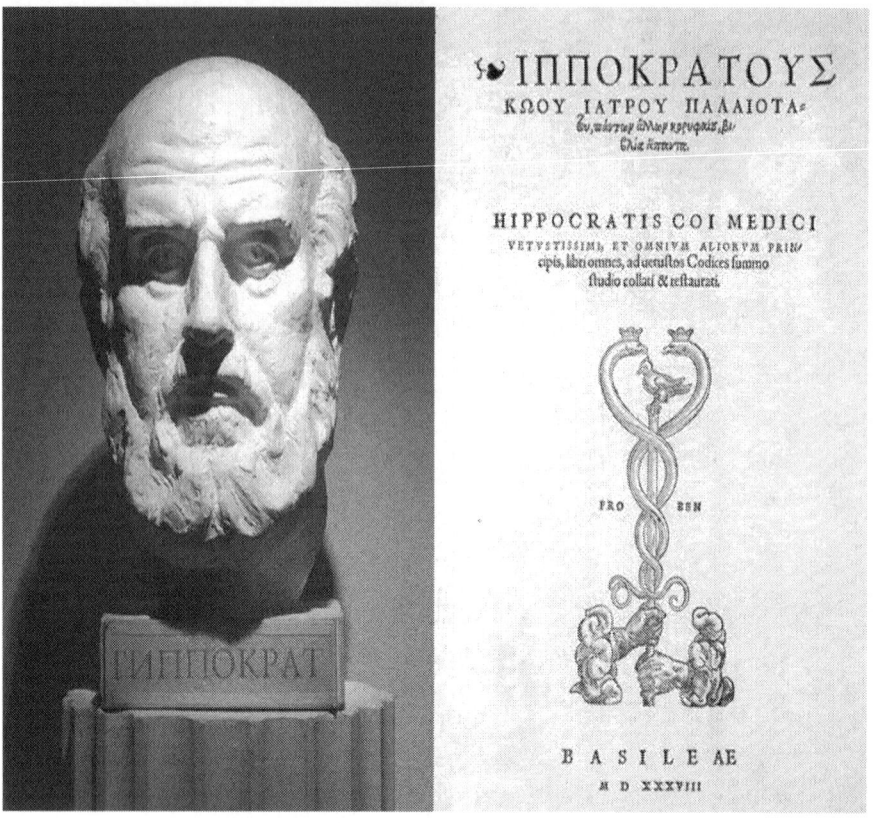

Hippocrates and one of his Books.

"As to diseases, make a habit of two things: to help, or at least to do no harm"   Hippocrates

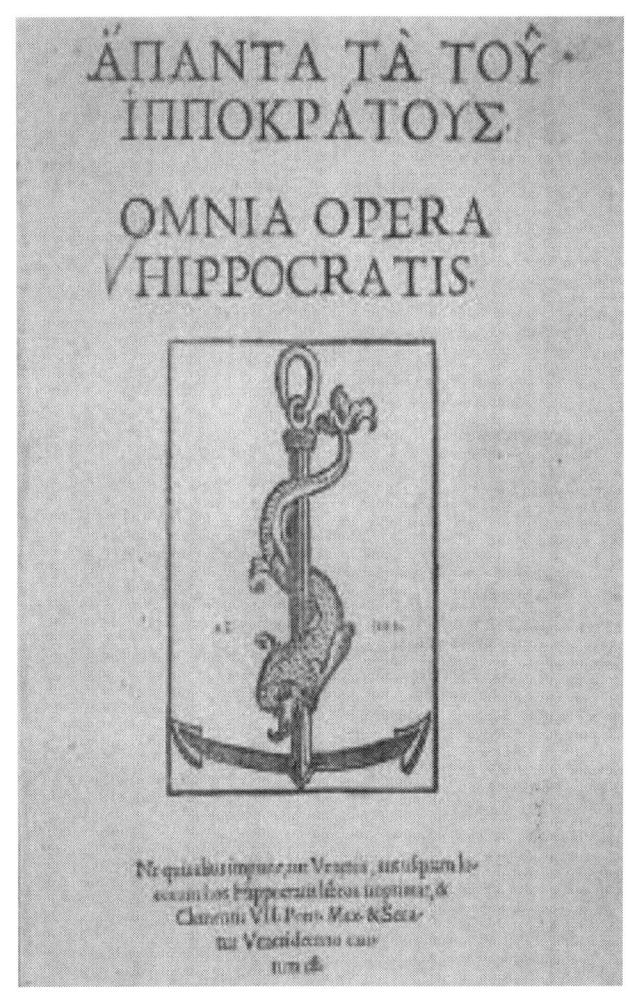

ÁΠΑΝΤΑ ΤΑ ΤΟΥ
ΙΠΠΟΚΡΑΤΟΥΣ

OMNIA OPERA
HIPPOCRATIS

Old writing of the Hippocratic Oath

The Egyptian book-loving Pharaoh Ptolemy 323-285 BC commissioned Egyptian scholars to collect and write down all of Hippocrates writings and teachings. They proceeded and wrote down every medical piece of information with Hippocrates name on it. Because of this, some of the current writings we have of Hippocrates are unlikely written by him.

Hippocratic Oath – Modern Version

I swear to fulfill, to the best of my ability and judgment, this covenant:

I will respect the hard-won scientific gains of those physicians in whose steps I walk, and gladly share such knowledge as is mine with those who are to follow.

I will apply, for the benefit of the sick, all measures that are required, avoiding those twin traps of overtreatment and therapeutic nilism

I will remember that there is art to medicine as well as science, and that warmth, sympathy, and understanding may outweigh the surgeon's knife or the chemist's drug.

I will not be ashamed to say "I know not," nor will I fail to call in my colleagues when the skills of another are needed for a patient's recovery.

I will respect the privacy of my patients, for their problems are not disclosed to me that the world may know. Most especially must I tread with care in matters of life and death. If it is given me to save a life, all thanks. But it may also be within my power to take a life; this awesome responsibility must be faced with great humbleness and awareness of my own frailty. Above all, I must not play at God.

I will remember that I do not treat a fever chart, a cancerous growth, but a sick human being, whose illness may affect the person's family and economic stability. My responsibility includes these related problems, if I am to care adequately for the sick.

I will prevent disease whenever I can, for prevention is preferable to cure.

I will protect the environment which sustains us, in the knowledge that the continuing health of ourselves and our societies is dependent on a healthy planet.

I will remember that I remain a member of society, with special obligations to all my fellow human beings, those sound of mind and body as well as the infirm.

If I do not violate this oath, may I enjoy life and art, respected while I live and remembered with affection thereafter. May I always act so as to preserve the finest traditions of my calling and may I long experience the joy of healing those who seek my help.

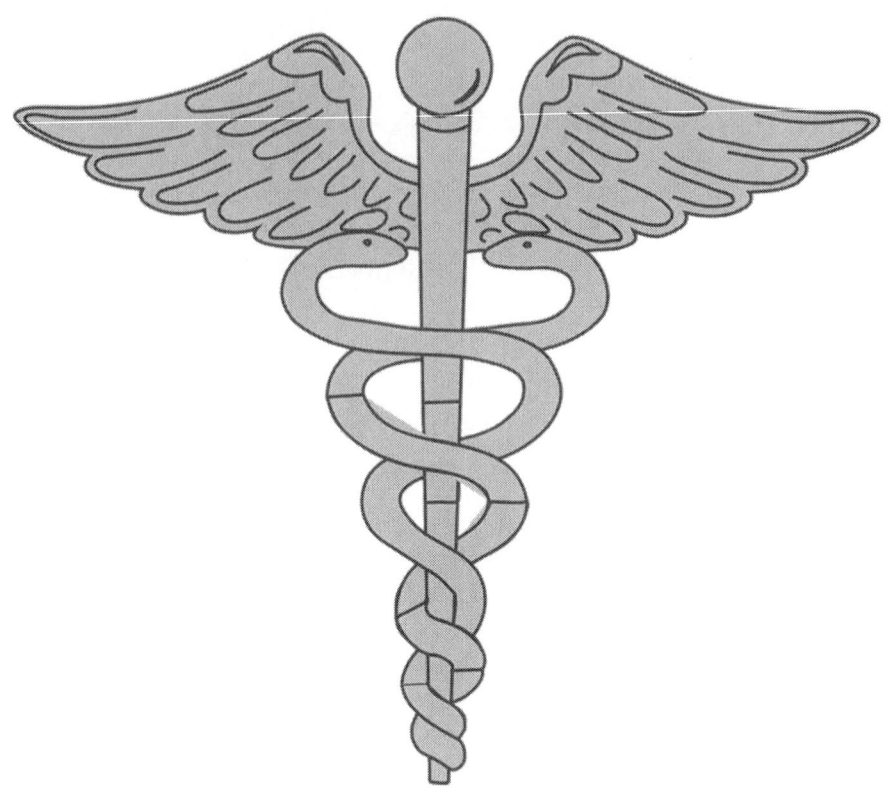

The staff and snake are still used as a medical symbol today.

In the Iliad, Homer mentions Asceplius, a skilled physician and the father of two Greek doctors in the city of Troy. The Rod of Asclepius became a Greek symbol of medicine, a serpent coiled around a rod. In ancient Greek religion and mythology, Asclepius was the son of Apollo

Moses is believed to have raised a serpent and put it on a staff, when bitten by the serpent, those who believed in god survived and those who did not were devoured by the serpent.

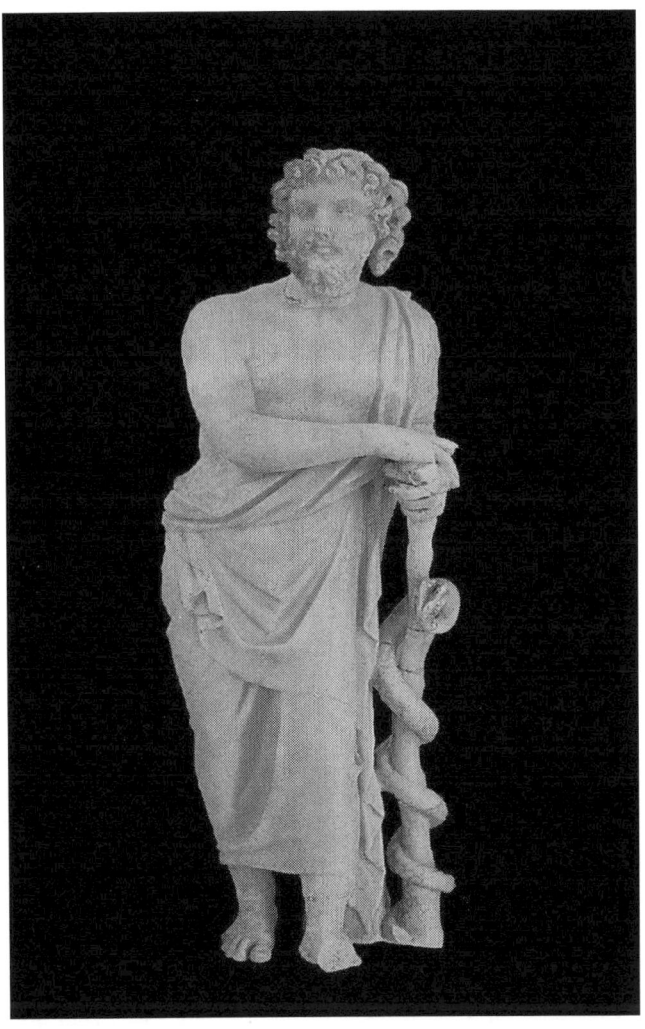

Asclepius was a mythical Greek hero and the Greek god of medicine and healing. The main attribute of Asclepius is a physician's staff with a snake wrapped around it. The staff and snake are called an "Aesculapian wand."

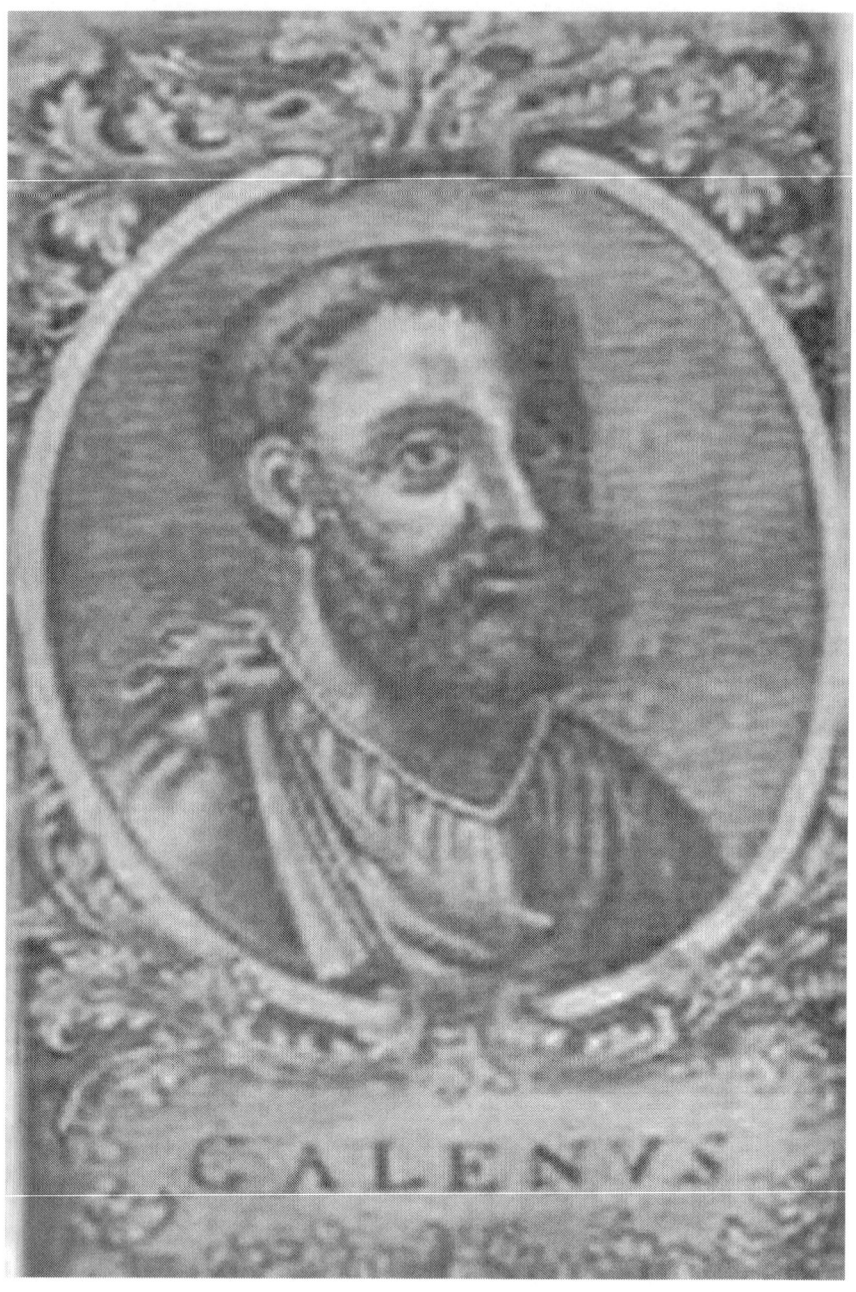

Galen

Galen (AD 130–200)

Clarrissmus Galenus of Pergamon was a great Roman physician, originally born in Greece. Galen completed his medical training at Smyrna. He wrote many books, including three on pulmonary diseases, one on ophthalmology, and another about the uterus intended for use by midwives. He traveled extensively in his career and is said to have maintained twelve scribes. In all, he wrote some 300 books, of which 118 volumes survived and eventually these were condensed down into 20 books.

After his training in Smyrna, he spent nine years traveling the known western world. While traveling, he expanded his medical education, diagnostic and treatment skills. His travels took him to Alexandria in Egypt, which boasted the largest library in the known world at that time. During his time period, some doctors traveled from city to city to see patients. He also traveled to Corinth, Crete, Palestine, and Phoenicia among his ventures, all of which were rich in medical information. After years of travel and working as a doctor, he was considered the most knowledgeable physician of his time.

He learned anatomy mostly from animal dissections, as human dissection was not an accepted practice until the Renaissance period. However, history books tell us Galen did do one human dissection on a man shortly after the man drowned. He dissected a hippopotamus, an elephant, and many pigs and monkeys. He believed the liver was the source of red blood cells and that it pumped blood to the entire body. (Of course we now know this is incorrect. It is the heart.) His understanding of anatomy and physiology were considered doctrine until the Renaissance period, some fifteen hundred years later.

Returning from his worldly travels, he became supervising physician to the gladiators in his native Pergamon. This provided him an opportunity to develop better treatments for human injuries. He improvèd techniques of splinting and bandaging wounds.

In the year 174 AD, Marcus Aurelius, the emperor of Rome, was returning from combat with the Germans, and he asked for Galen's consultation. By querying and appraising the "imperial fever," Galen diagnosed an upset stomach and recommended the equivalent of a warm-water bottle be applied to the emperor's abdomen. Marcus Aurelius agreed with the diagnosis and gave Galen great praise for his acumen as a physician. From that moment on, Galen was to enjoy great popularity and an abundance of patients seeking his services.

During his lifetime, Galen became famous as a doctor and popular for his beneficial therapies. Patients sought and wrote for Galen's consultations from areas as distant as Spain, Gaul, and Syria. After curing a woman of melancholy, he received four hundred gold pieces. He discovered that injury to the laryngeal nerve caused aphasia. After examining a patient with numbness in his hands, Galen was able to attribute the symptoms to an old neck injury, this highly impressed the patient. He made medicines himself and held contempt for charlatans who "falsified or made poor medicines." Galen's reputation and the number of his followers flourished.

The Galenic teachings and writings of medical treatment dominated medical teaching and treatment for the next fifteen hundred years. In fact, little at all changed during the Dark Ages, and no attempt was made to improve medical therapy for 15 centuries. In many circumstances, it regressed. New ideas were not even considered, as Galen's writings were felt to be doctrine in European medicine.

Although many of his therapies were beneficial, many were not effective but used anyway. Not until the Renaissance, a time of enlightenment, was Galen's ideas of medicine challenged.

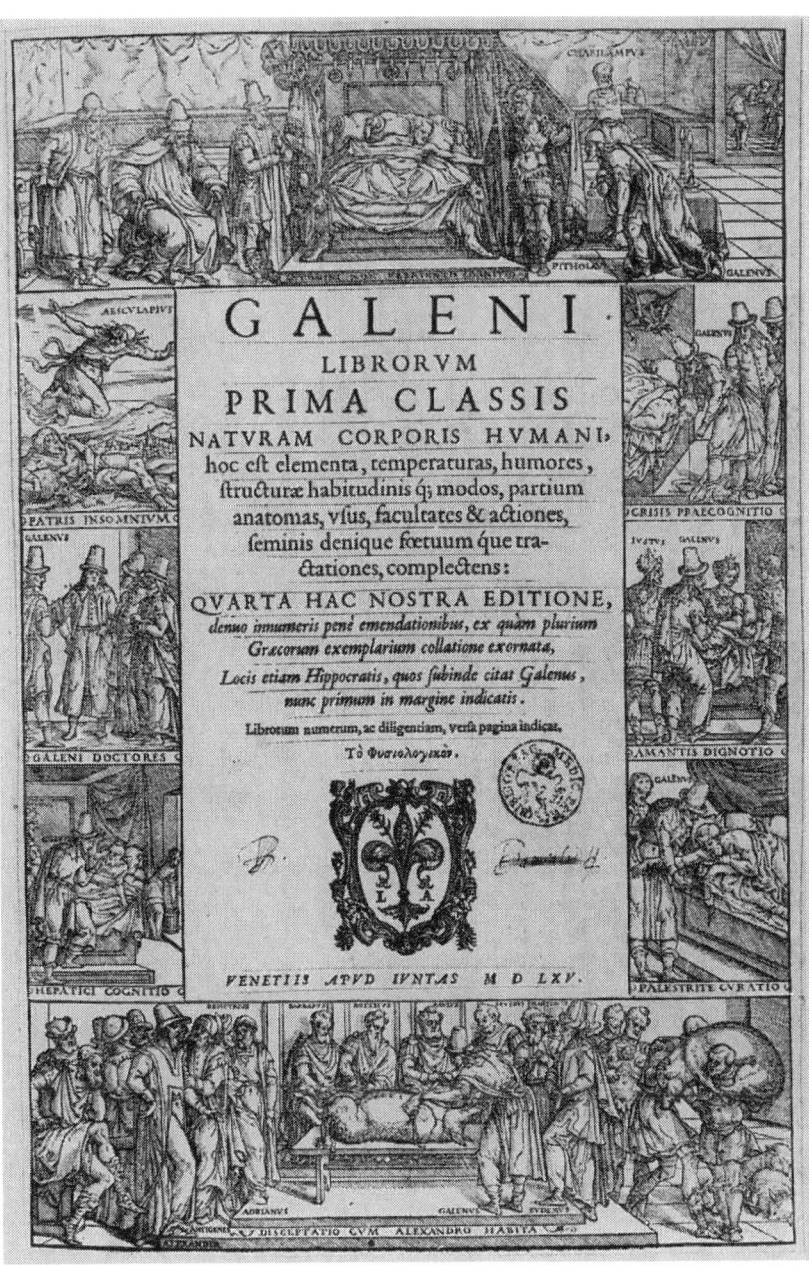

Cover of book of Galen's teachings

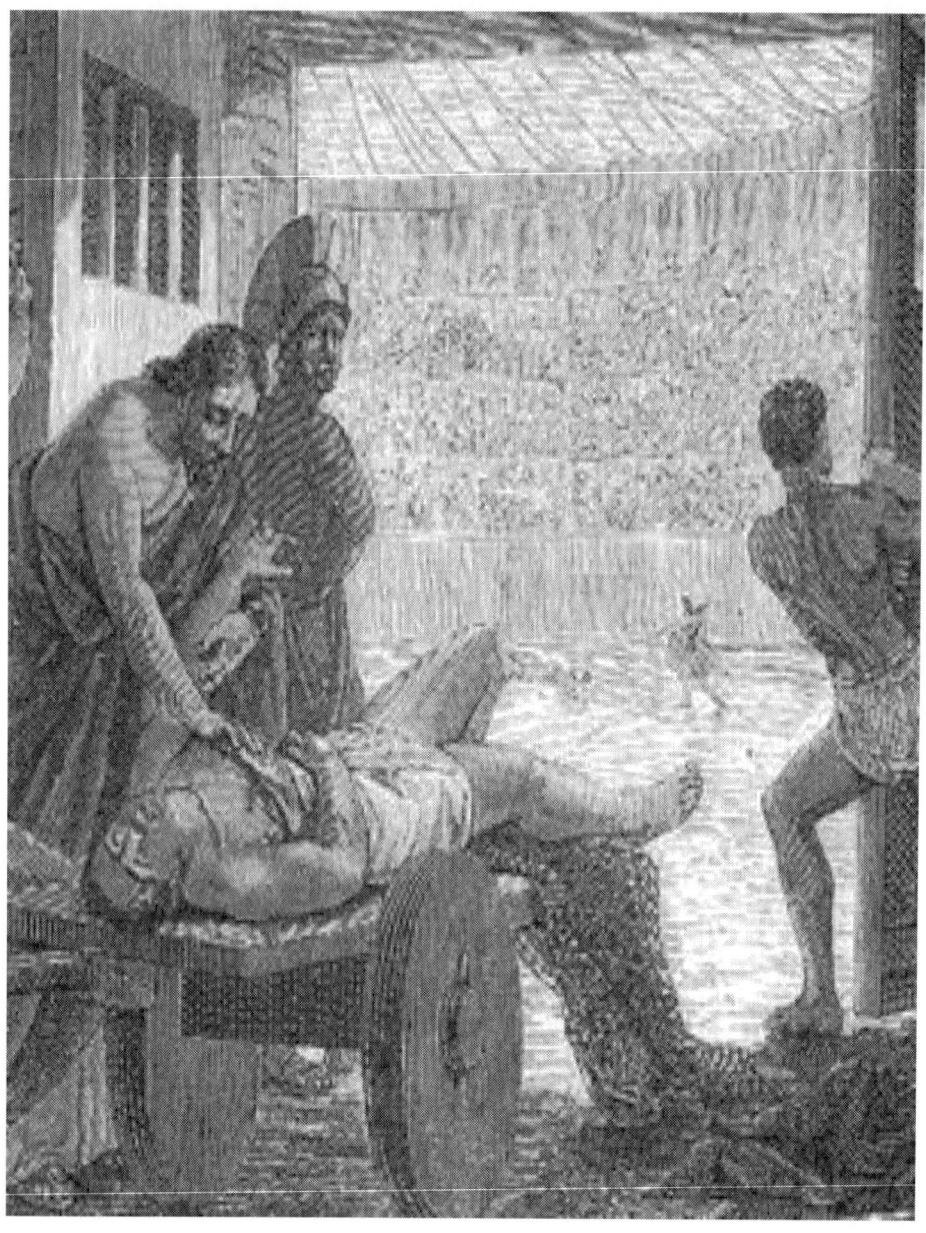

Galen traveled extensively and at age 28 became medical supervisor of the gladiatorial amphithear in his home town Pergamon.

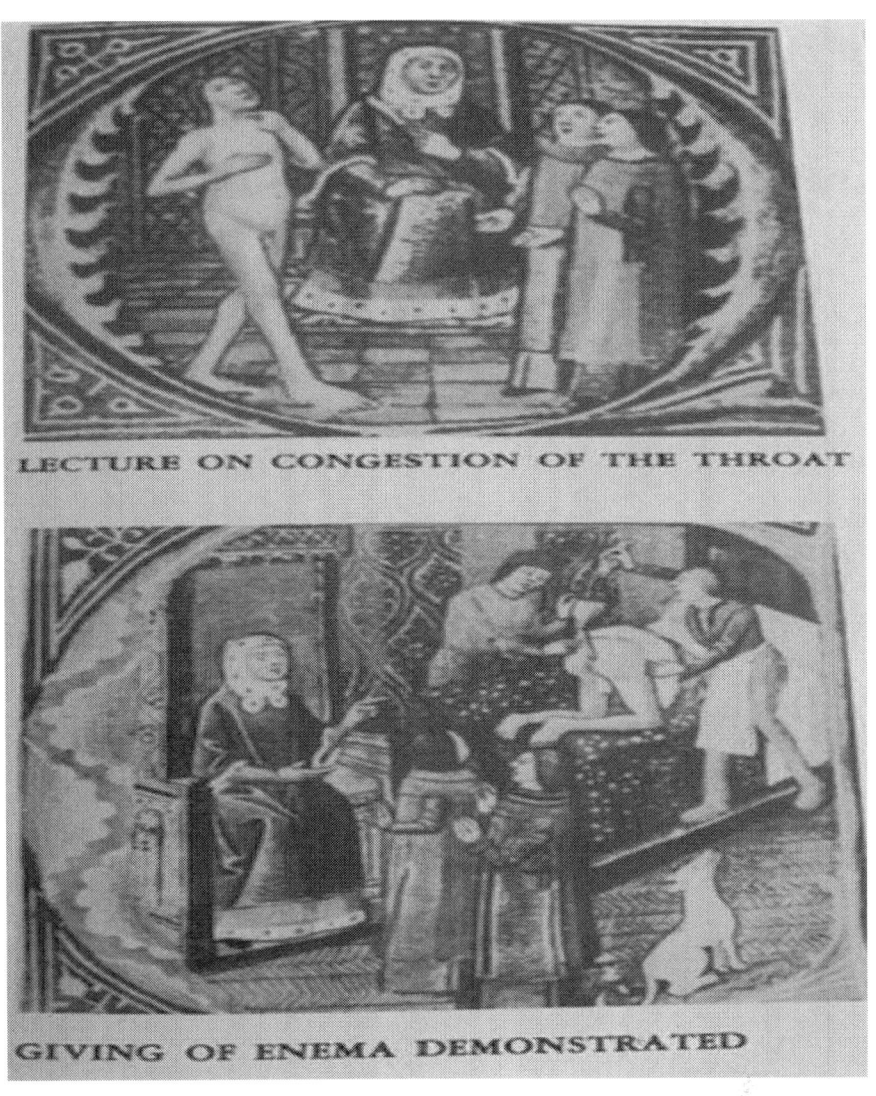

LECTURE ON CONGESTION OF THE THROAT

GIVING OF ENEMA DEMONSTRATED

Drawings from Dresden Galen manuscript (15th century) Throat pain and constipation, Galen's teachings provided answers.

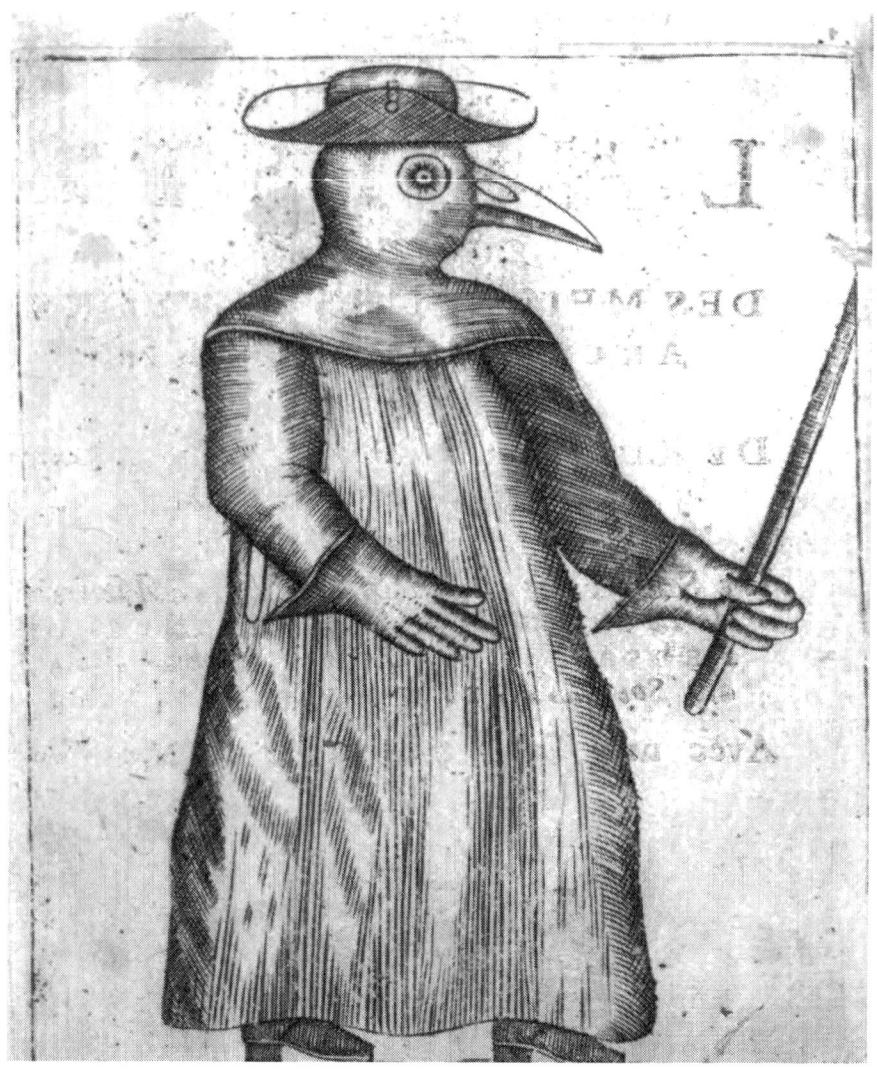

Black Death Doctor in Personal Protective Garb
This was developed in the 17th century primarily to fight off the smell when near the dead, and maybe prevent getting infected if near a patient with bubonic plague.

The Black Death – bubonic plague

Although Roman and Venetian physicians wore similar outfits since the 14th century, the **plague doctor costume** became widespread in France in the 17th century. It is credited to the French doctor Charles de Lorme in 1656.

Doctors wore a mask with a beak often filled with sweet or strong smelling substances, often including lavender. This was to defend against the putrid smell of dead bodies. They also wore gloves, boots, a wide-brimmed hat, eye coverings, and an outer over-clothing garment to protect themselves (much like the modern day personal protective equipment worn treating patients with infectious dieaseases). The plague caused by the bacteria Yersinia Pestis, was carried by fleas from rats.

Some historians estimate the pandemic that ravaged Europe between 1347 and 1351 killed over 200 million people, over four years!

In 541 BC the plague was in Constantinople, and from there spread to to Europe, Africa, and Aisia killing from 30-50 million people, at the time about half of the world's populatoin.

Until the identification of the bacteria Yersenia Pestis, and antibiotics, was the plague eventually, a little but a minor medical problem. Current antibiotics prevent futher outbreaks. At the times of the plague, germ theory was not known, and neither was a bacteria or virus. Still people understood that getting close to someone with the plague was a common way to catch it themselves. Doctors were often helpless and often caught the plaque and succumbed to it when they came in contact with it's victims.

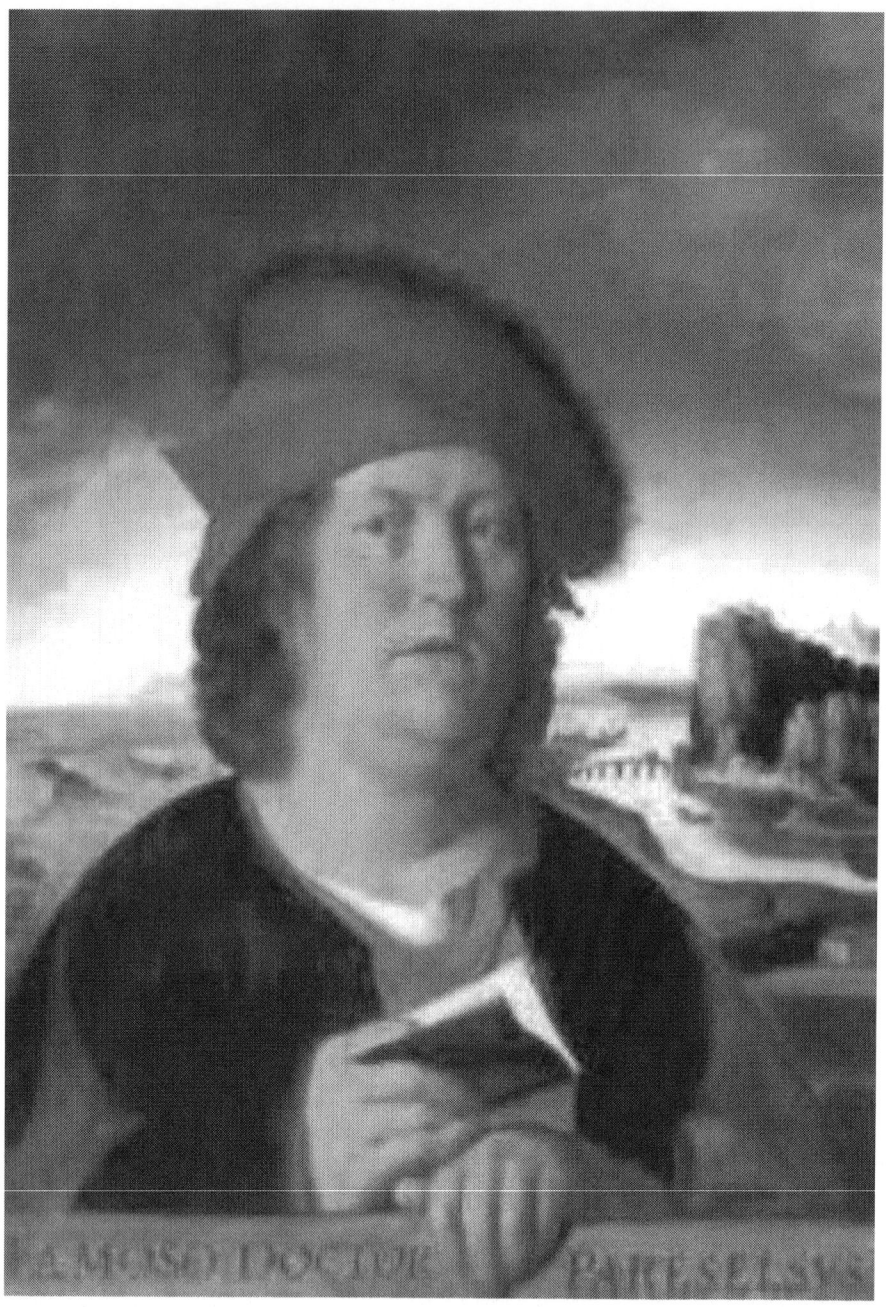

Paracelsus

Paracelsus (1493–1541)

Paracelsus was the first to significantly change medical thought since Galen. Paracelsus has been called the founder of medicinal chemistry, and was known for his elaborate details describing mental illness. He was famous for beginning a lecture series by lighting a huge fire and throwing the works of Galen into it. This was his way of saying, "Let's take it from the top." He believed Galen was a liar and a faker.

Paracelsus entered the University of Basal in 1507, but he disliked the teachings. After attending eight different universities, he received his degree from Leonicenus in 1516. He had a strong belief that a doctor must be a traveler because *experience is knowledge.* He used the first known chemical medicines, including mercury compounds. Paracelsus also discovered sulfuric ether for anesthesia (but did not use it on people), and he understood the association between environment and disease. Specifically, he wrote and described *black lung* in coal miners.

Perhaps his most important work was his documentation of various mental diseases. He believed that man was composed of antagonistic animal and godly spirits, which Freud later elucidated as the id and superego. Paracelsus was noted to say, "You should treat the spirit, for it is the spirit that here lies the sick." He believed lack of faith could create disease—and cure some as well.

In contrast to Hippocrates, Paracelsus was intensely concerned with himself as a legate of God, the supreme physician. Preoccupied with eternity and the soul of man. He felt that a physician was neither a pill maker nor businessman. His perfect physician was a philosopher, astrologer, alchemist, and above all, a virtuous man. Paracelsus proclaimed the character of the physician was far more effective in curing illness than skill.

Paracelsus was not generally well accepted during his lifetime. However, after his death, his work laid a foundation for new thought, and a new bravery to question the old teachings of Galen. He opened the doors, inspiring curious physicians to further study new therapies and progress for both physical and mental illness.

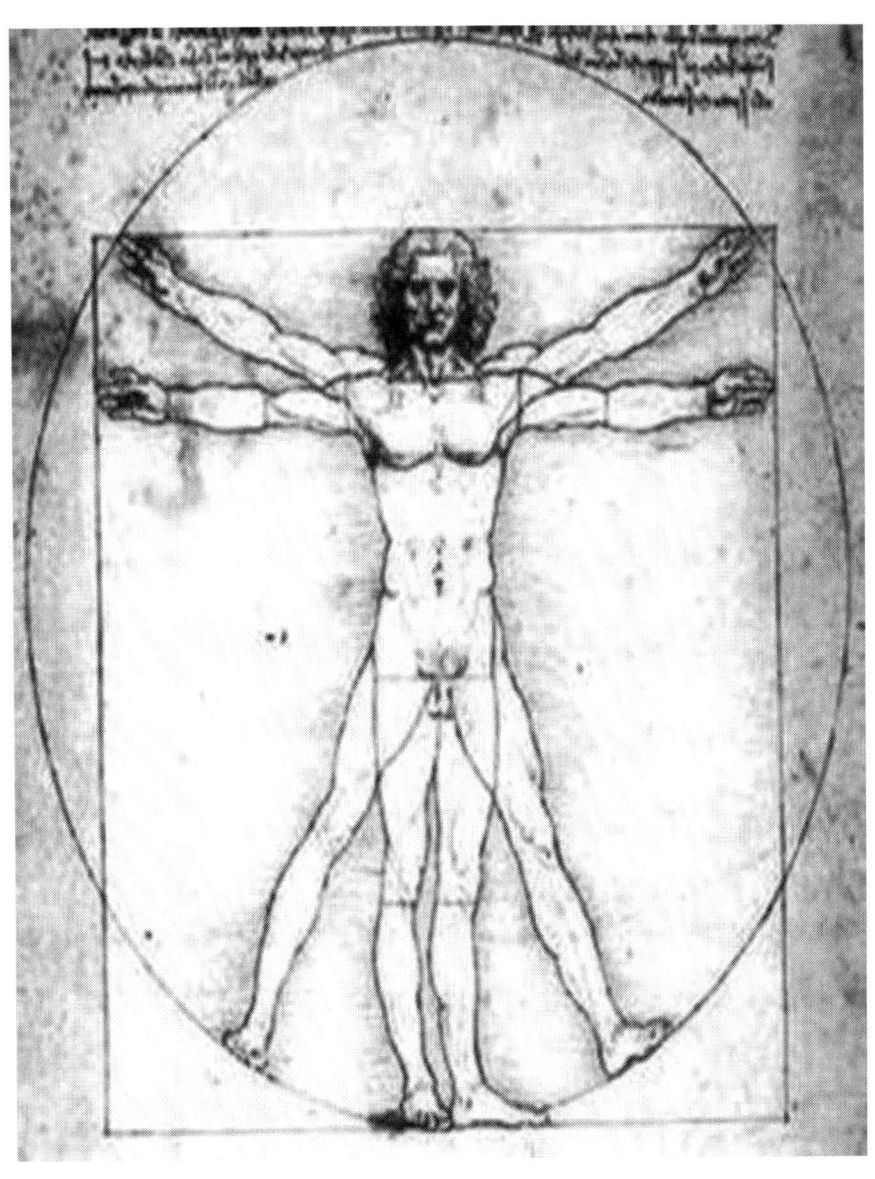

Leonardo Da Vinci's drawing of Vitruvian
man with dimensions, *c.* 1487.

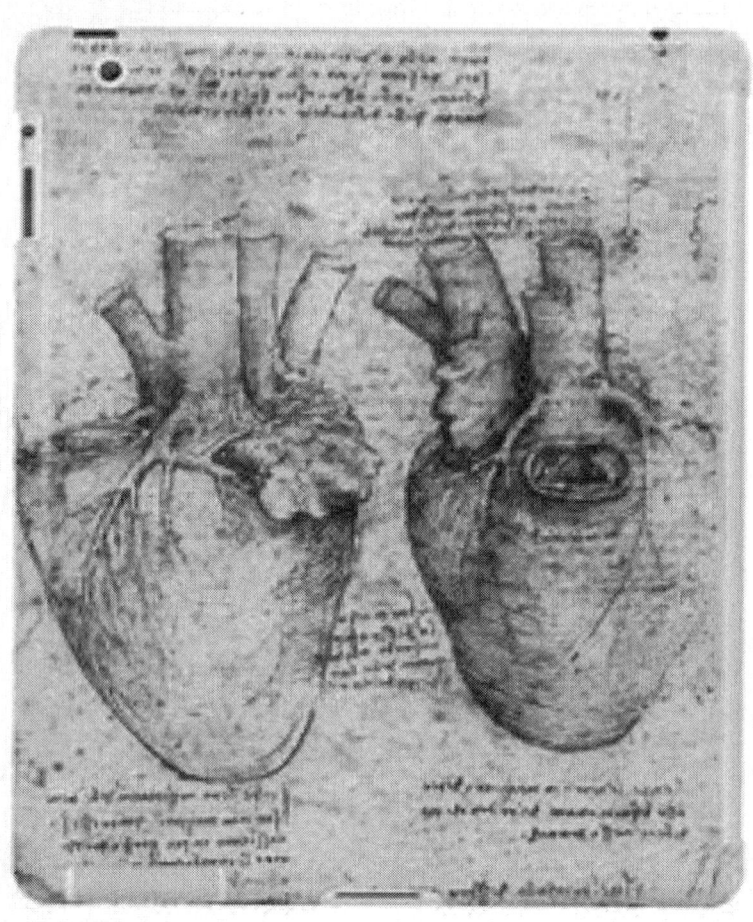

Leonardo da Vinci's sketch of the human heart. c. 1508. His drawings were remarkably accurate and advanced anatomical studies better than any time in the history of medicine. He helped advance medicine, although he never trained as a physcician.

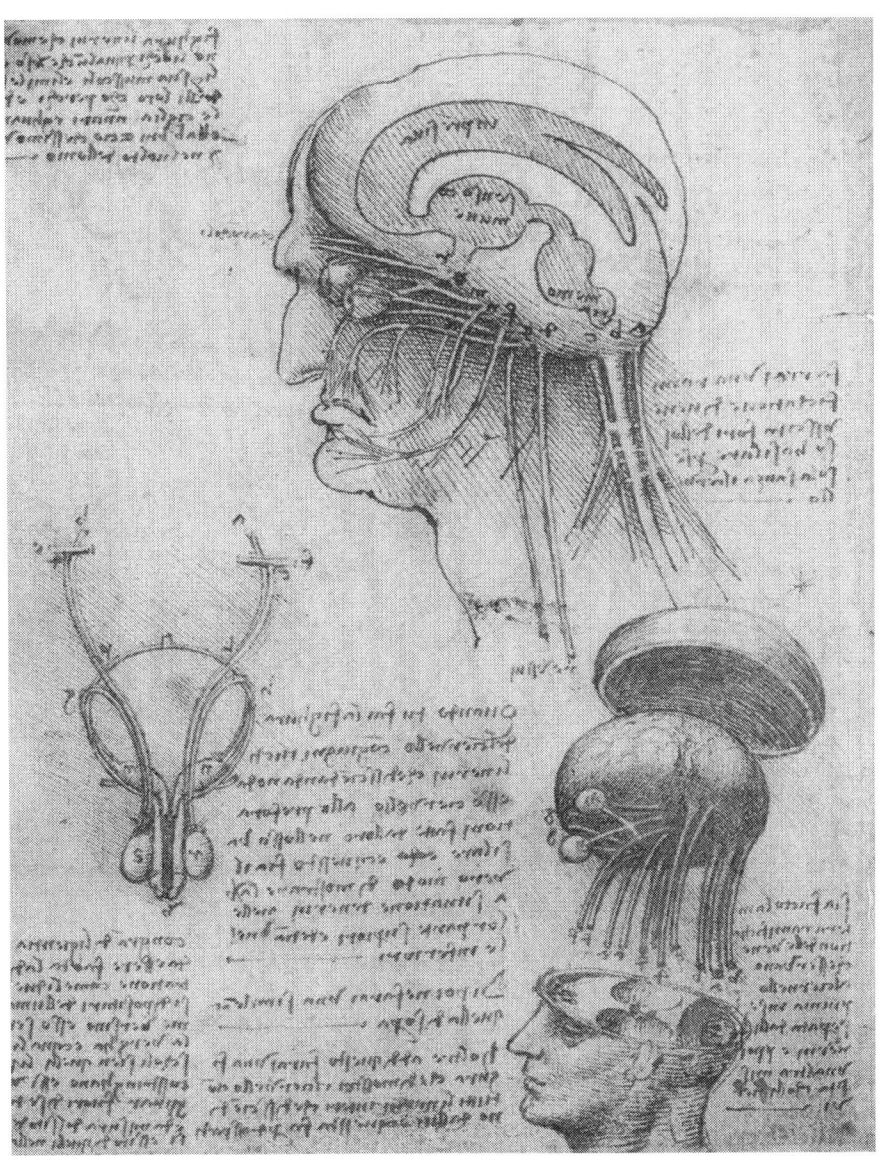

Leonardo da Vinci draws the human with adept details, and is able to dissect bodies illegally at first. Eventually he got special permission from the catholic church to dissect and sketch what he learned for a medical book.

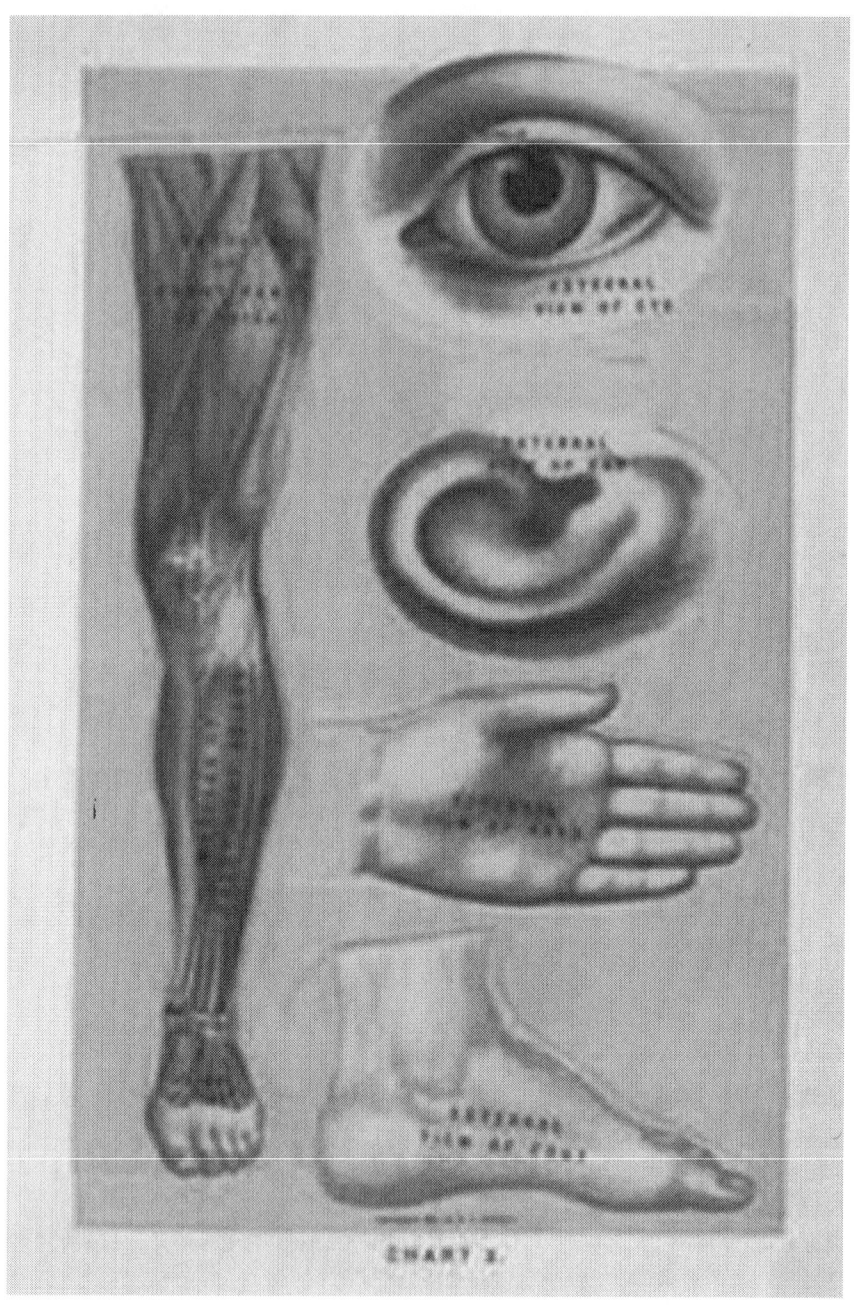

Some of Leonicenus Drawings

Leonicenus (1421–1524)

During the rebirth period of the Renaissance, exploration of forgotten doctrines was reopened and explored. Leonicenus played a large part in translating Latin works of Pliny's Natural History, printed in Venice in 1469. Pliny the Elder was a Roman scholar who wrote and encyclopedic *Natural History* in the first century AD, a body of work that like Galen survived and was an authority on scientific matters through the Dark Ages.

In 1492, Leonicenus published his own revolutionary work with his book entitled *Concerning the Errors of Pliny and Others in Medicine.* The translation of Pliny's work and in-depth clarification and editing by Leonicenus on medicines derived from plants, animals, and minerals gave rise to modern botany and pharmacology.

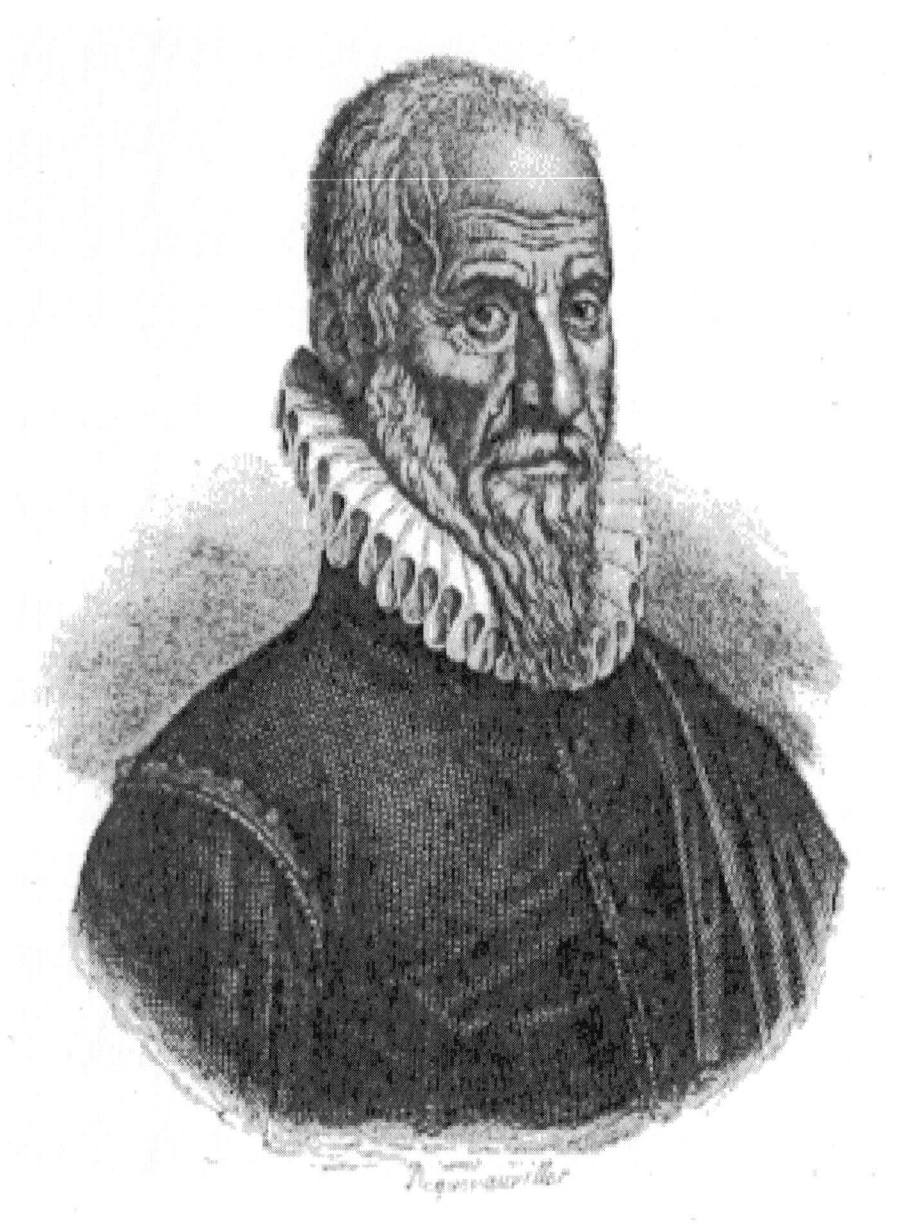

Ambroise Paré

Ambroise Paré (1510–1590)

The pure science of human anatomy has little effect on a patient until a physician uses the knowledge for practical purposes. Ambroise Paré helped join the science of anatomy with the art of medicine.

Barbers were the surgeons in the fifteen hundreds, and Paré apprenticed with one. After an apprenticeship, he studied at Hôtel-Dieu in Paris and became a military surgeon. On the battlefield, wounds were usually cauterized with scalding oil or a hot iron. At one point, his regiment ran out of scalding oil. Paré improvised and used a type of ointment that actually aided in healing instead of destroying tissue by burning it. In 1545, he published his findings and helped change wound treatment thereafter. He also found that chopped raw onions and salt were helpful for severe burns.

Between 1545 and 1550, he worked at College Saint-Côme in Paris, where he developed practical manuals for surgical treatments. This was in contrast to many of the pure anatomy texts of the day. He was a central figure in binding the science and observation of anatomy that Vesalius studied, to its practical usage in treating patients.

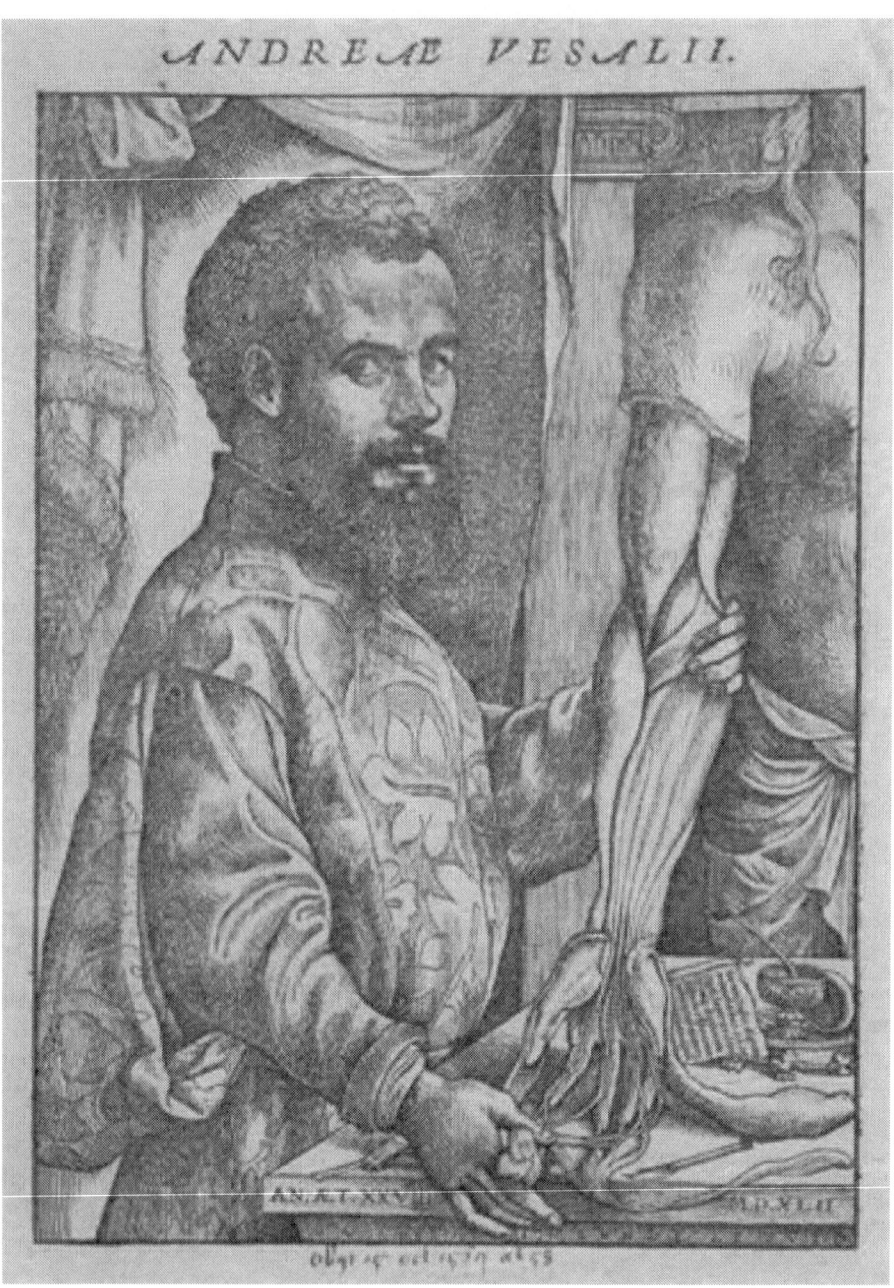

Vesalius

Vesalius (1514–1564)

As Paracelsus opened the doors to the pursuit of new scientific exploration, others like Vesalius were needed to do the footwork. The study of cadavers was accepted during the Renaissance period. After meticulous study, Vesalius wrote *De Humani Corporis Fabrica*, seven books on the structure of the human body. This was the first complete textbook on anatomy, and for the first time, a significant fusion between science and medicine occurred. The precision of his drawings made Galen's followers soon accept Vesalius's human anatomy as more useful and practical.

Vesalius was soon acknowledged as one of the foremost physicians in Europe. He founded his own successful private practice and sold medical information in the form of health charts. These were in high demand during the sixteenth century. For a time he was court physician to the Holy Roman Emperor Charles V and physician to King Philip II of Spain— both very prestigious positions.

Andreas Vesalius was born in Brussels and died on the island of Zante after a shipwreck on the voyage home from a pilgrimage to the Holy Land.

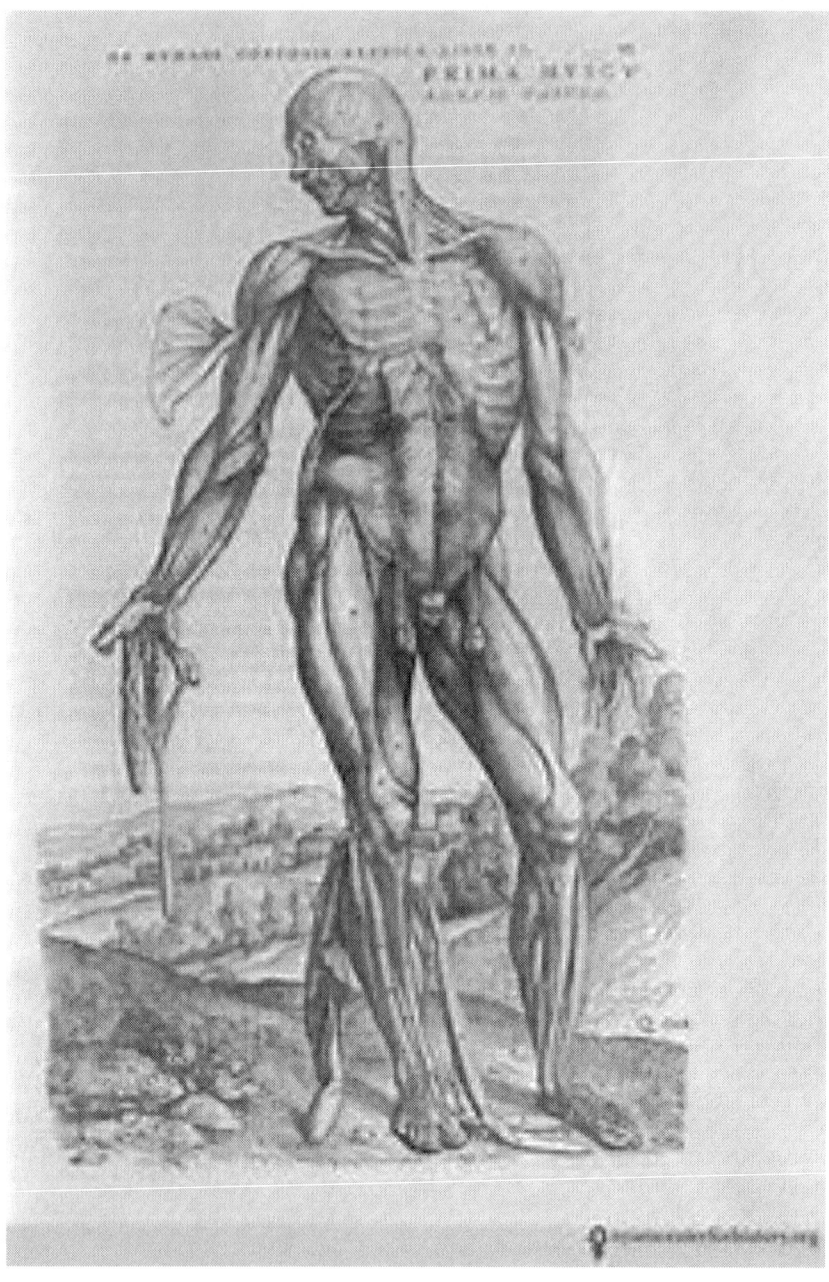

Vesalius was one of the first to dissect and draw the human body in detail. Here is a fontal view of the body by Vesalius in the 1500s

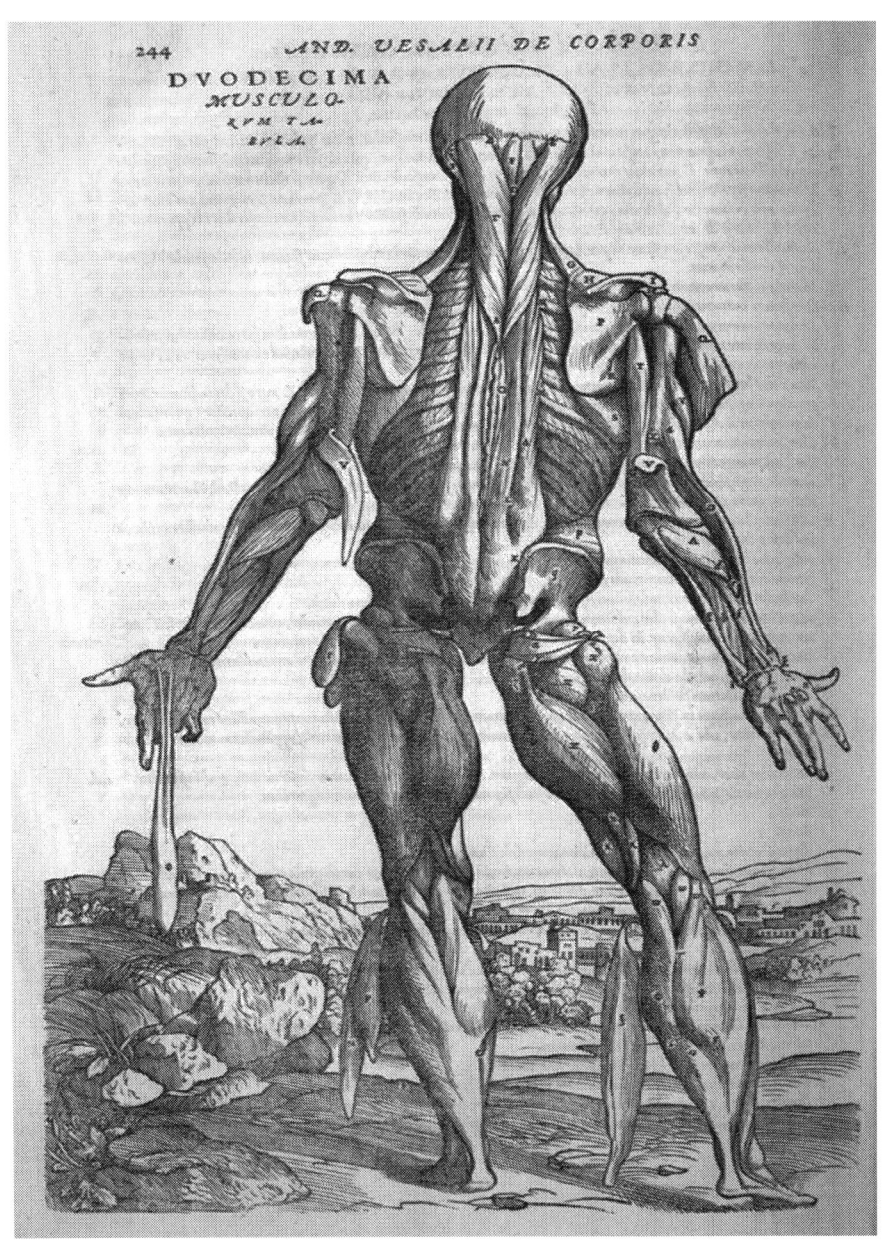

Drawing of the back muscles by Vesaliu

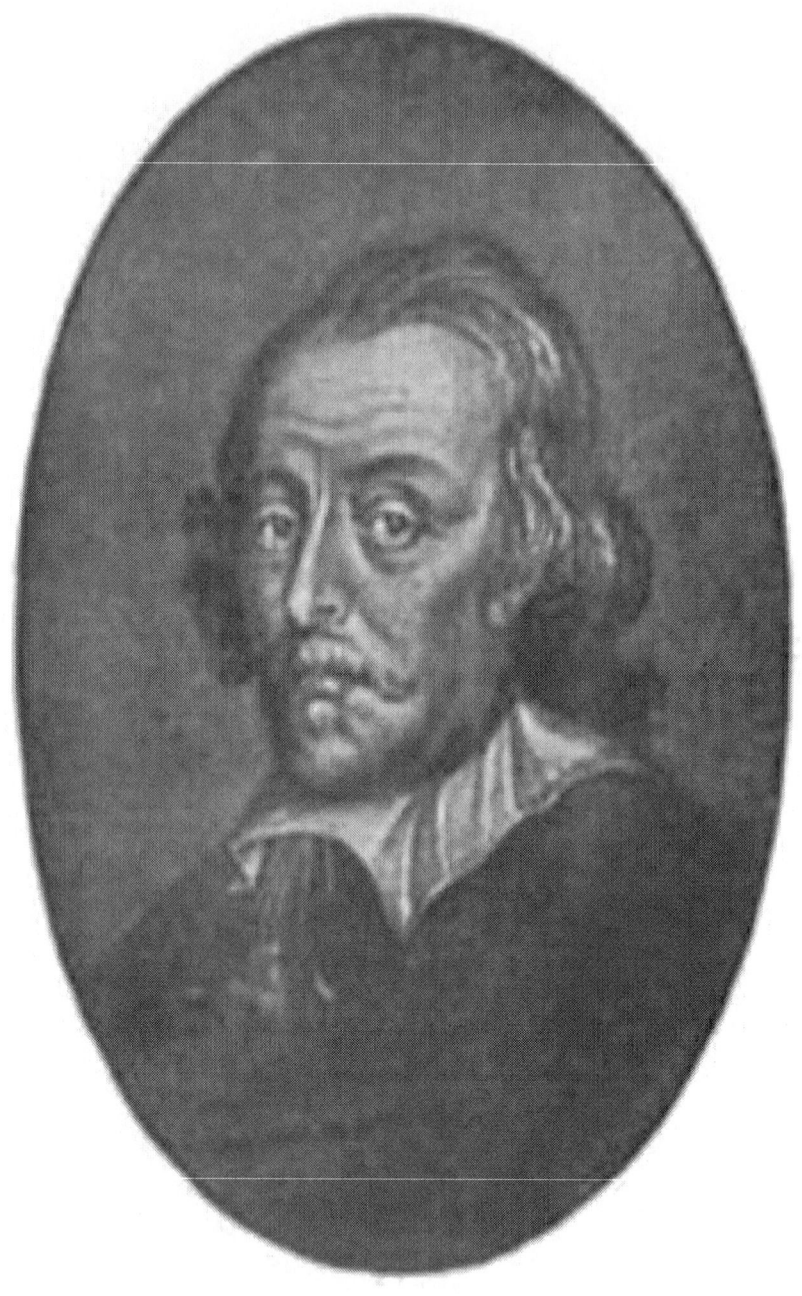

William Harvey

William Harvey (1578–1657)

The relationship between the heart, blood vessels, and pulse took William Harvey twenty years of research to figure out correctly.

According to the teachings of Galen, it was still believed for over a thousand years, that the liver pumped blood through the circulation. Harvey published his conclusions in Latin in *Exercitatio Anatomica de Motu Cordis et Sanguinis in Animalibus* ("On the Motion of the Heart and Blood in the Animal") in 1628. This was the single most convincing evidence that experimental physiology was a valuable tool in medicine. This novel experimental work proved that all of what Galen wrote could be subject to study in an objective manner through research and the scientific method.

Harvey attended college at Cambridge and then earned his medical degree in Italy. His later studies and experiments were to change how the medical community viewed the human circulation right up to modern times.

In Padua, Harvey studied under Fabricus, who himself was the successor to Gabrielle Fallopia (after whom Fallopian tubes are named). Fabricus learned from his own studies on veins that these vessels had one-way functioning valves, an insight that aided Harvey's correct understanding of the circulatory system. Harvey knew from his own studies that with each heartbeat a pulse was felt. In experiments, he observed that a heart slows prior to death, and with this slowing, so does the pulse. Blood, he correctly reasoned, must be pumped from the heart. But which vessels in the circulation go in which direction? Given that veins have one-way valves, allowing blood only to move in the direction of the heart, he therefore concluded correctly that the arteries receive the pulse and blood first. He then deduced that blood "must pass through some pore returning to the veins, to the vena cava, and finally to return to the heart," and thus he predicted the existence of capillary pores.

Harvey's conclusions, it is interesting to note, were published and titled *De Motu Cordis*, which is a seventy-two-page, five-and-a-half-by-seven-and-a-half-inch volume, of which some fifty-five original copies were made. Each today is worth in excess of $300,000.

Harvey also spent much time studying reproduction. His work *On Generation*, described the embryos of chickens, which laid the foundation for the study of embryology.

The relationship between the heart, veins, and arteries was solved. But the scientific community balked at Harvey's conclusions. His private practice suffered because of the criticisms he received. Over the years, however, his model of the circulation was finally accepted as fact. The scientific community was slow to accept change. In fact, he would have presented his studies earlier, but without substantial scientific evidence, he risked being ostracized from the medical community.

In subsequent years, when other physicians were finding Harvey's conclusions correct, both Harvey's reputation and practice grew. After which, he became a well-acclaimed and sought-out physician. He became so well acclaimed that he became physician to King James I, Charles I, and the lord chancellor, philosopher, and statesman Francis Bacon. Interestingly, Frances Bacon's philosophical ideas supported the scientific method, which was not well established at the time.

In his later years, William Harvey had gout, which caused him great discomfort. He retired honorably from the Royal Society of

Physicians. At the age of eighty-three, he suffered a stroke and died shortly thereafter.

During William Harvey's era and the renascence, the age of reason sprouted and new discovers and improvements in medicine were making progress and moving doctors away from Galen's teachings. For the first time, a significant and monumental contribution in medicine was fueled by the efforts of experimentation.

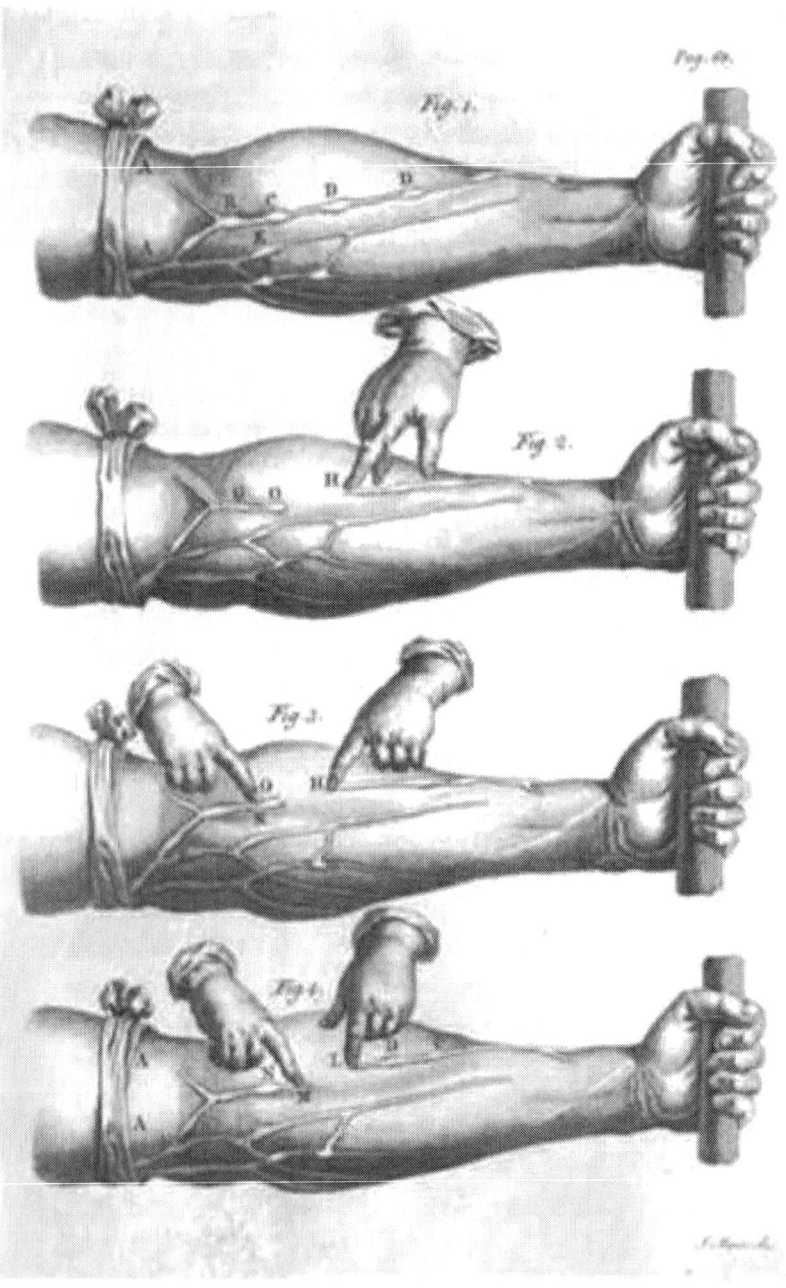

William Harvey's picture on circulation

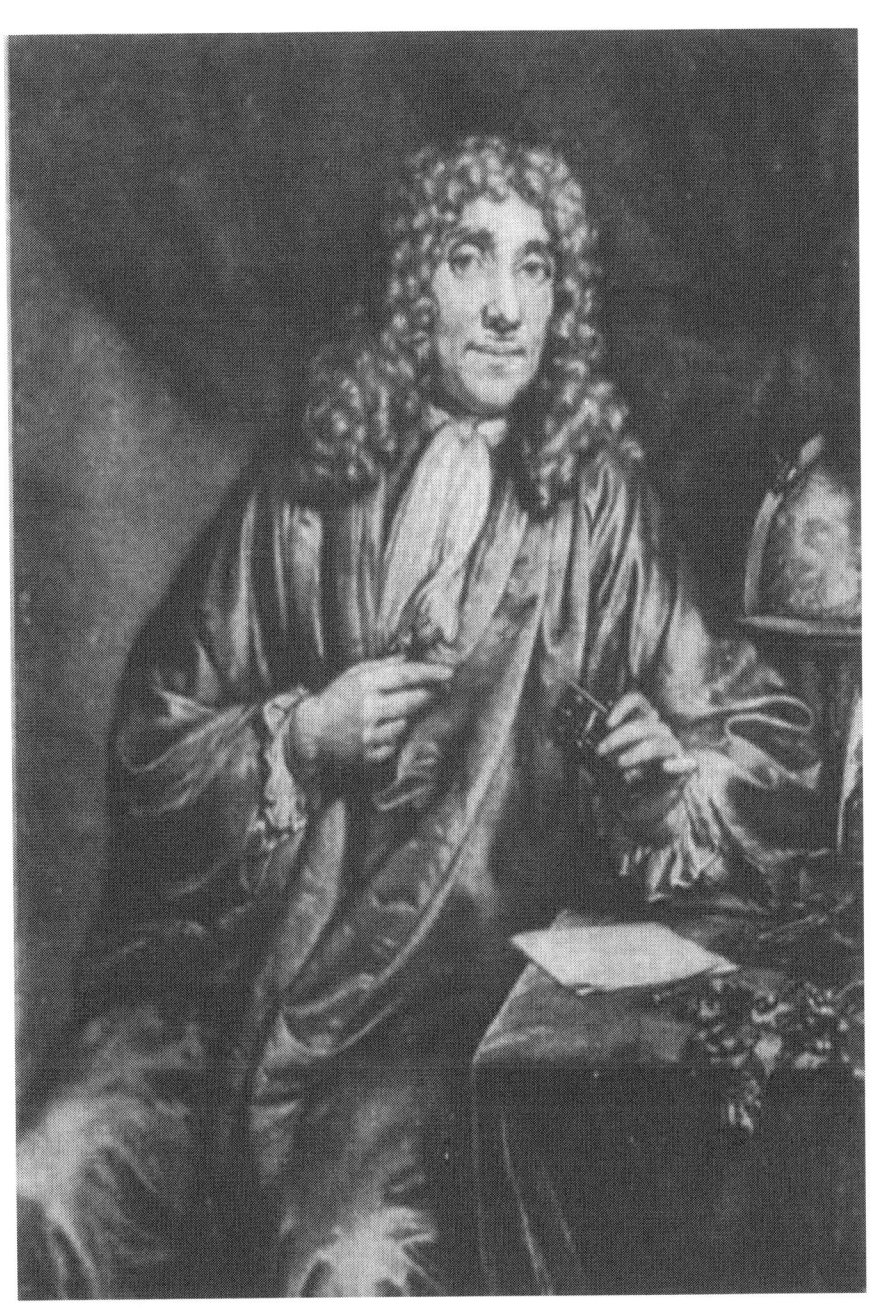

Antony van Leeuwenhoek

Antony van Leeuwenhoek (1632–1723)

Van Leeuwenhoek was a Dutch merchant who never left his homeland. He began as a cloth merchant and then later worked in the construction of microscopes. He built a total of 247 microscopes in his lifetime and discovered that he obtained better results using a single short-focus lens, unlike other microscopes in common use during his studies.

He conducted much of his work secretly in his native Dutch town. Starting in 1673, he began sending papers to the Royal Society in London. With his microscopes he discovered protozoa, made careful descriptions of red blood cells, illustrated and described spermatozoa and the structure of yeast, and made accurate descriptions of the life cycles of fleas, ants, and weevils. The first microanatomy was described by van Leeuwenhoek, with observations and descriptions of blood vessels, eyes, muscles, nerves, skin, and teeth.

This merchant who was never trained as a physician was the first to describe the microbial world. Although it took until the nineteenth century to make the connection between bacteria and infectious disease, van Leeuwenhoek is credited as the father of microbiology and protozoology.

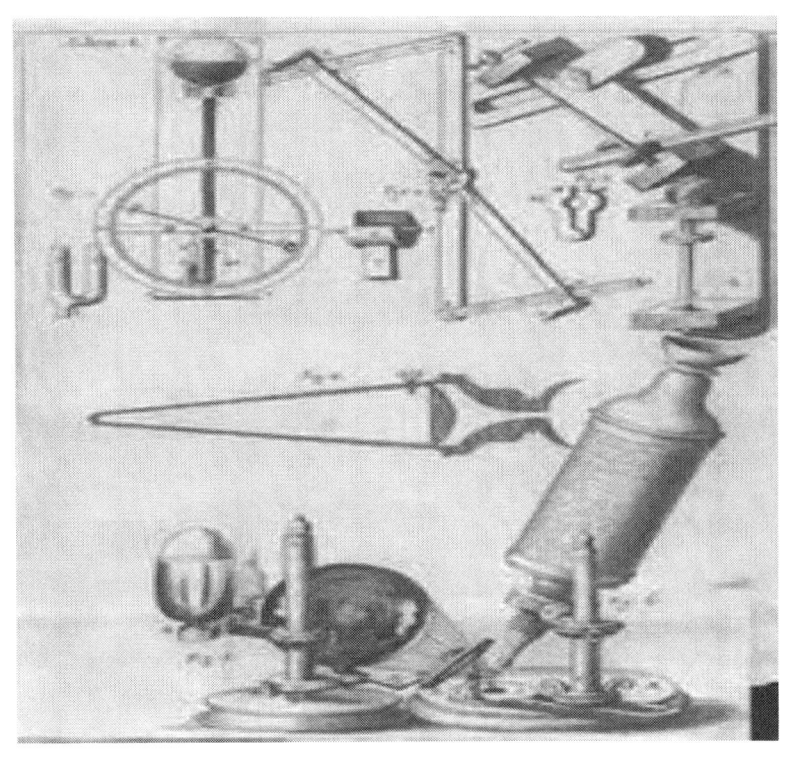

Old microscope

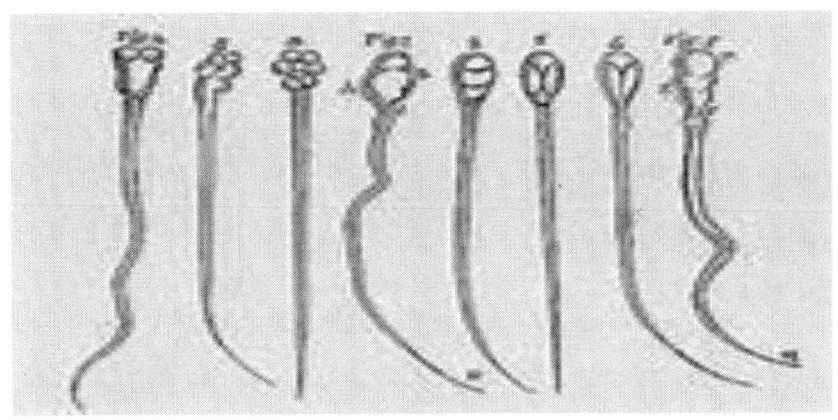

Old Drawings of sperm

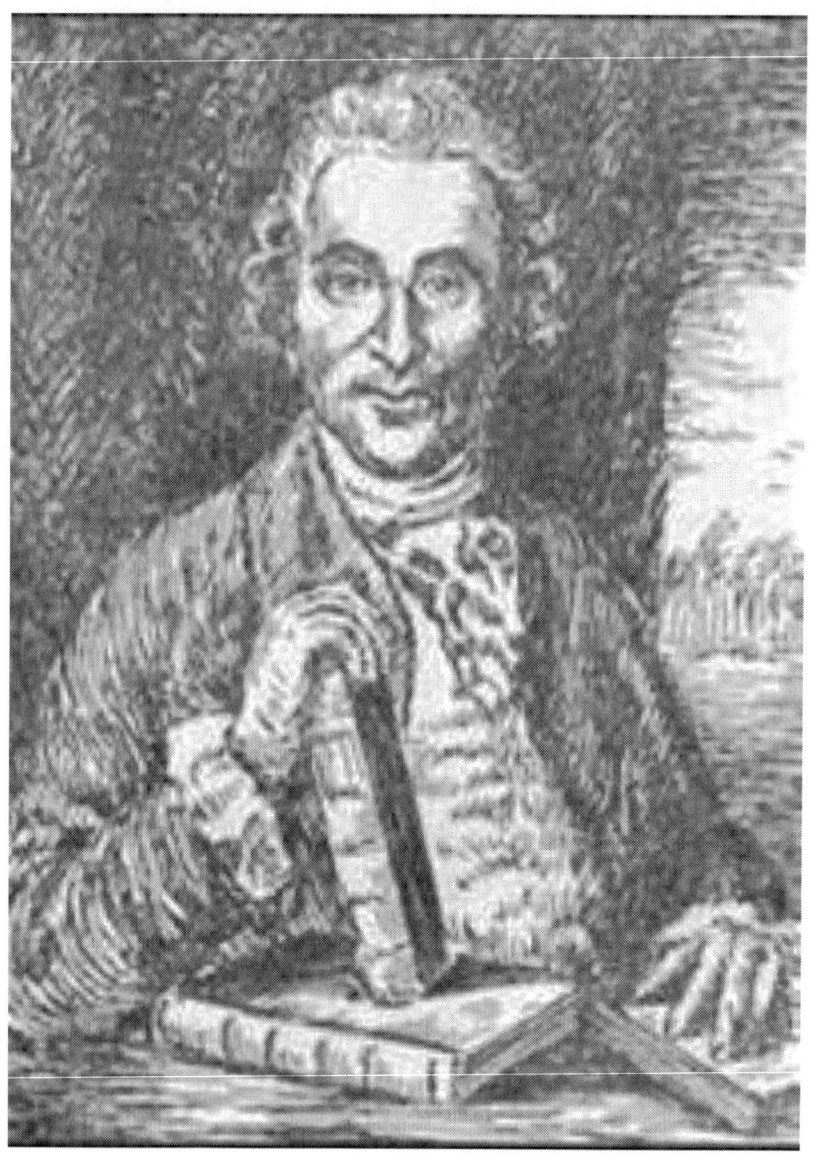

James Lind

James Lind (1716–1794)

For years, scurvy was a dramatic and fearful disease, especially for sailors on long voyages. In the early seventeen hundreds over a third of the sailors with Vitus Bering, who sailed to discover the western coast of America, died of scurvy. The world would not remember Bering or the strait that bears his name at all had his crew not eaten berries while shipwrecked on an island. It was felt that a limited diet contributed to scurvy. But it wasn't until 1753 until James Lind did his experiment with sailors, was there a known cure and prevention of scurvy discovered.

Lind guessed that scurvy was caused by a faulty diet. He did an experiment with twelve sailors who had acquired scurvy on a sailing voyage. To two of those affected with scurvy, he gave lime juice, and they promptly returned to duty. The remaining ten sailors went on to further suffer the scourge of scurvy. In his *A Treatise of the Scurvy*, Lind recommended citrus and vegetable foods in the diet of sailors. This won him international acclaim, even though the Royal Navy in England was slow to adopt his proposals. However, one year after his death, the British government adopted the policy of using these foods on all sailing ships. This adaptation helped maintain the health of Captain Cook's crew as he sailed around the world from 1768–1771. The English naval men were nicknamed "limeys" after their widespread use of fresh fruits and vegetables, which included drinking sips of lime juice.

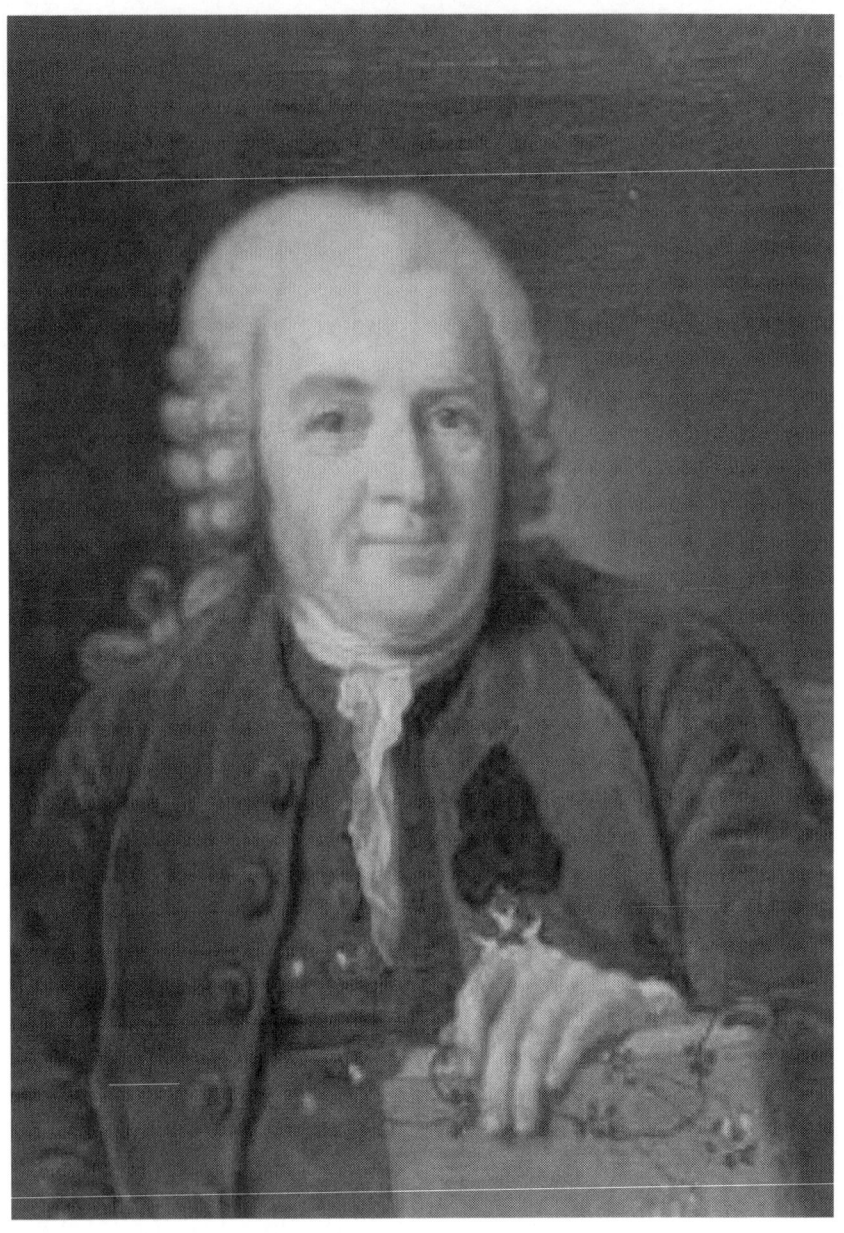

Carolus Linnaeus

Carolus Linnaeus (1707–1778)

Linnaeus wasn't sure if he wanted to become a botanist or a physician. Born in Sweden, he studied botany and earned a medical degree. He was very interested in the classification of plants, and while studying for a time in Holland, he published three books: *The Fundamental System of Nature in Botany*, *General Plants*, and *The Flora of Lapland*. For the first time, Linnaeus classified organisms by their reproductive similarities. He divided plants into classes, which he then subdivided into orders, families, genera, and then species. In all he published some 180 works, classifying animals, minerals, and plants. Taxonomy is the name given to classifying plants and animals. It is interesting to note that Charles Darwin's *Origin of Species* was written in 1859 and likely used Linnaeus ideas of classification in developing his theories of evolution.

Linnaeus's classification system won universal acceptance, and students flocked from all over Europe to hear him lecture. He received a Swedish knighthood in 1761, and the system of classifying plants today is basically the same as when Linnaeus classified them some 250 years ago.

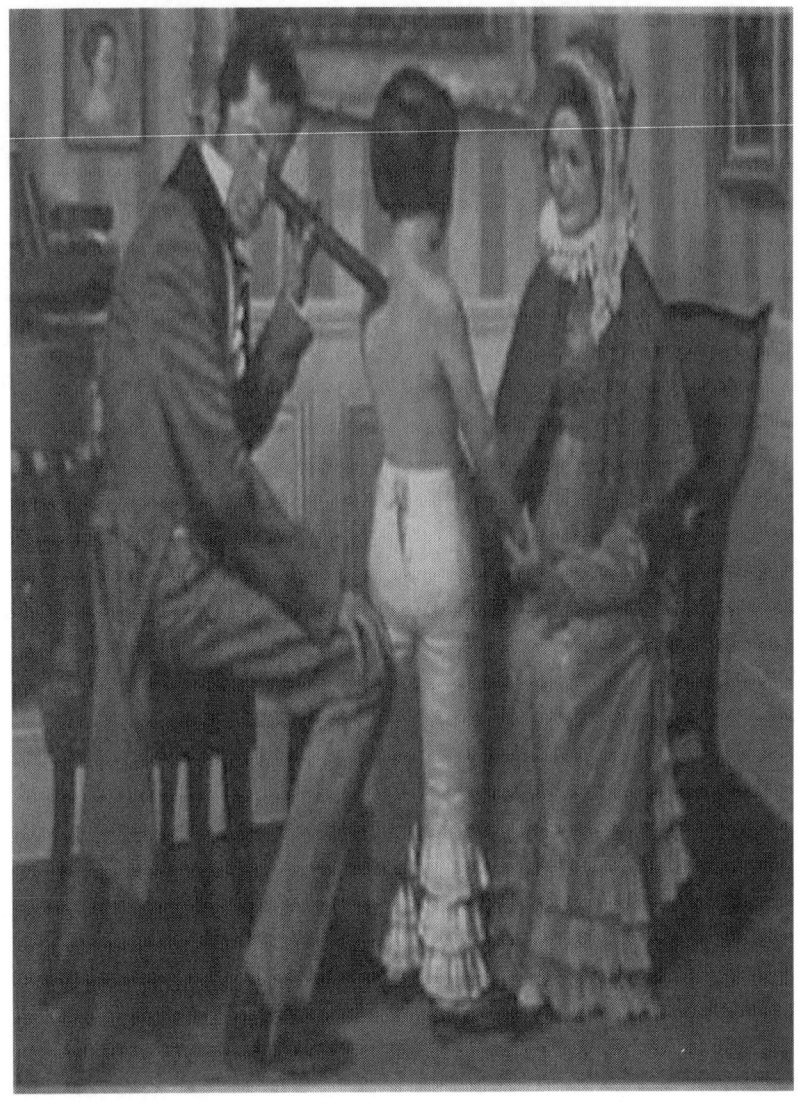

Rene Laennec

Rene Laennec (1781–1826)

Laennec received his medical degree from the School of Medicine in Paris. He became editor of the prestigious *Journal of Medicine*, but what he is most remembered for is his invention of the stethoscope.

Listening to the hearts of men was a simple matter. A physician would simply lay his ear against the patient's chest. Listening to the heart of a woman, on the other hand, was not considered acceptable. Laennec developed a hollow tube that, when one end was placed against the chest, allowed a physician to put his ear to the other end and listen to the patient's heart. This new invention, the stethoscope, helped maintain the proper respect toward female patients.

He died in 1826 of tuberculosis.

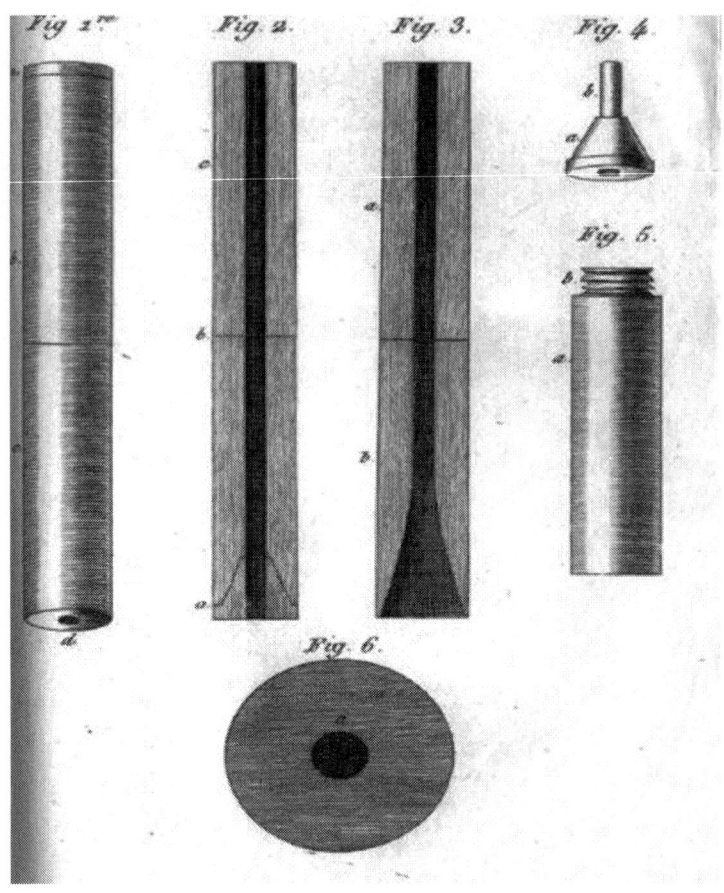

Drawings of Laennec's stethoscope. He invented it in the year 1816.

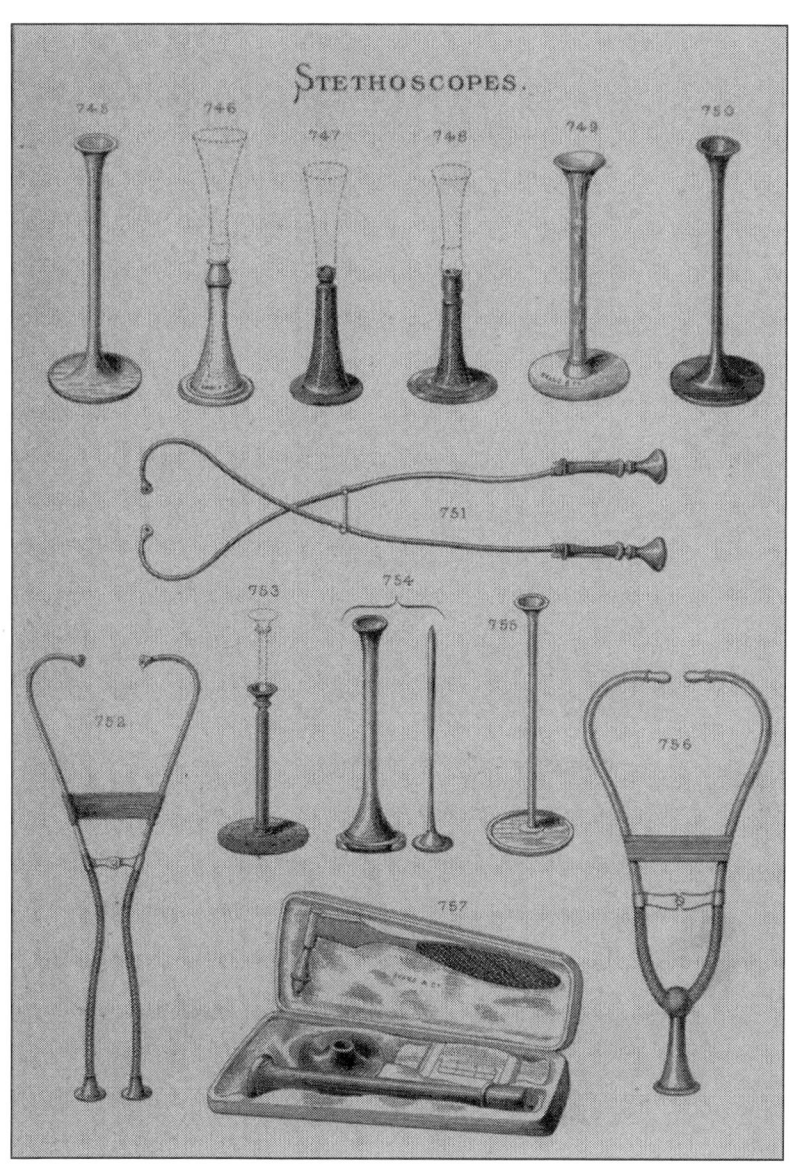

Evolution of the stethoscope

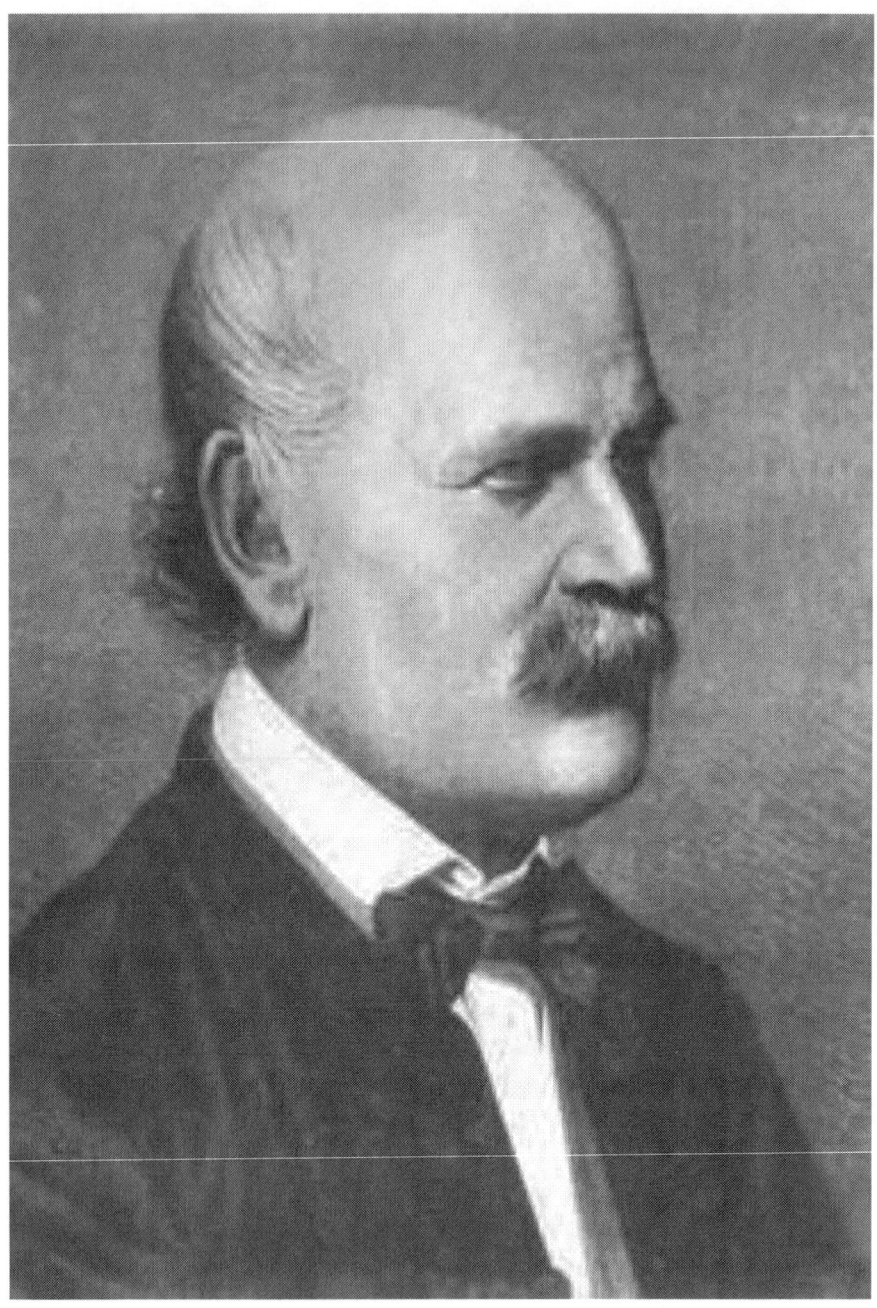

Ignaz Semmelweis

Ignaz Semmelweis (1818–1865)

Semmelweis was a hero in the fight against infectious diseases, although his life ended tragically. His observations as the first assistant at the Maternity Hospital in Vienna in 1847 led to a consciousness of handwashing as a way to prevent the spread of disease. He observed, that it was all too frequent, that after medical students and physicians dissected cadavers, then went to examine pregnant women, these women commonly got infections. These infections, called puerperal fever, carried with them a high mortality rate. Midwives' patients, however, at that time had a very low incidence of puerperal fever, as midwives did not examine cadavers prior to working on the maternity wards and delivering babies..

Puerperal fever often appeared following childbirth. Usually, it involved a bacterial infection of the endometrium, the lining of the uterus, caused by the bacteria *Streptoccocus pyogenes*. Since antibiotics were not available then, and germ theory wasn't understood until Louis Pasteur, sepsis ensued, and many women died shortly after childbirth.

Semmelweis was puzzled by the cause of puerperal fever. One of his favorite professors, Professor Kolletschka, died after a laceration he sustained while dissecting cadavers. The laceration became infected and then caused the professor to get septic and die. Semmelweis explained his observation twelve years later in an excerpt from his book: Kolletschka's…septic changes…arose from the inoculation of cadaver particles, then puerperal fever must originate from the same source…The fact of the matter was that the transmitting source of the cadaver particles was to be found on the hands of the students and attending physicians."

Semmelweis did not publish his findings soon after his discovery in 1847. He did present them, but only after his obstetrical position in Vienna was terminated in the middle of the controversy his conclusions stirred. In May 1850, three years after his initial observations, Semmelweis presented his conclusions at the Medical Society of Vienna. Although some physicians accepted his arguments, many still did not.

Semmelweis left Vienna in 1850 to enter the University of Pest in Hungary, and he eventually received a professorship. Not until ten years later, in 1860, did he eventually publish his discovery, entitling it *The Etiology, the Concept, and the Prevention of Puerperal Fever*.

Still, there was opposition to his theory that cadaver particles caused puerperal fever and that handwashing with chlorinated lime juice prevented it. He sent letters to obstetrical professors everywhere, explaining the importance of handwashing and his conclusions.

In July 1865, Semmelweis was having mood swings and memory problems and perhaps had become frankly psychotic. Some feel this was secondary to the rejection and stress of promoting his ideas. In a letter to Josefs-Akademie at the University of Vienna, Semmelweis wrote, "I bear the knowledge that since 1847, thousands and thousands of puerperal women have died…and would not have if I had not kept silent…And you, Herr Professor, have been a partner in the massacre. This murder must cease…In order to put an end to these murders, I have no recourse but to mercilessly expose my adversaries." Semmelweis was admitted to an asylum in Vienna. Two weeks later, he died there. He was forty-seven years old.

An autopsy presumably showed Semmelweis to have died from a laceration on his hand—and thus possibly from the same disease he attempted to battle against for over a decade. But this fact is debated.

Others speculate that syphilis or an early form of Alzheimer's disease caused his death. Perhaps the most plausible explanation was the beating he received in the asylum that attempted to control his psychosis. Some sources suggest that in all likelihood, he was beaten to death.

As Pare' did the footwork to help transfer Vesalius's anatomical studies in the laboratory to practical use for physicians taking care of patients, Ignaz Semmelweis started doing the footwork for the germ theory before it was even discovered. Louis Pasteur, several years later, was to discover bacteria as the causative pathogens in many diseases. Then Lister was to initiate further measures to develop antiseptic surgical techniques to prevent bacterial infections. Semmelweis's conclusions were a leap ahead. And still today, when examining patients, we hear his conscience stating, "Wash your hands."

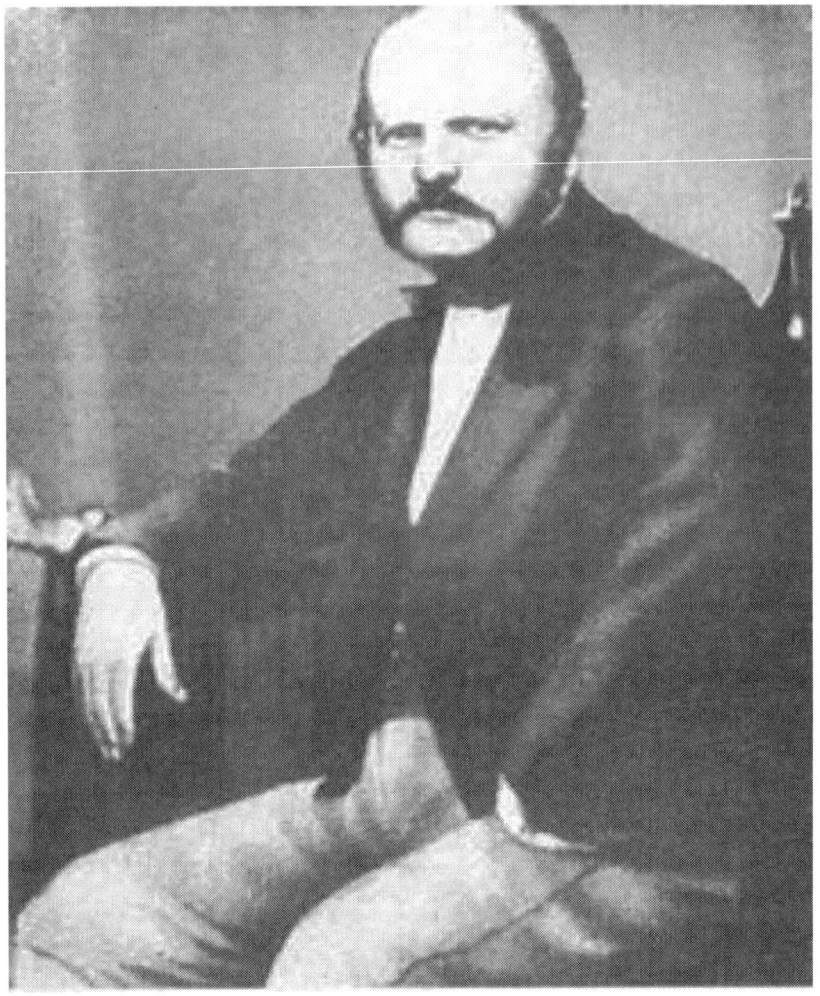

Ignaz Simmelweis c. 1857

He was the first to raise consciousness about hand washing, although severely criticized for it at the time. It may have even cost him his life.

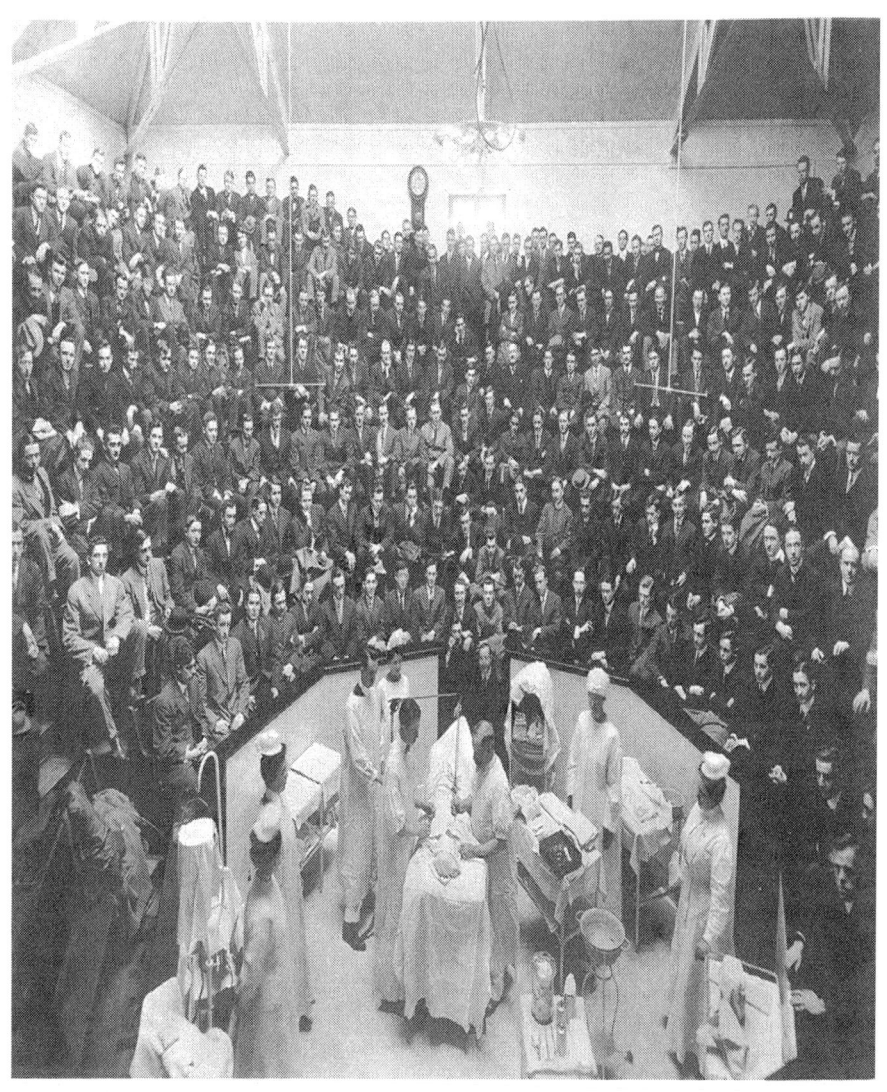

One of the ealry operating theaters was thought to be the 1804 operating theatre at the Pennsylvania Hospital in Philadelphia. Students and doctors would watch and learn as surgeons carried out operations.

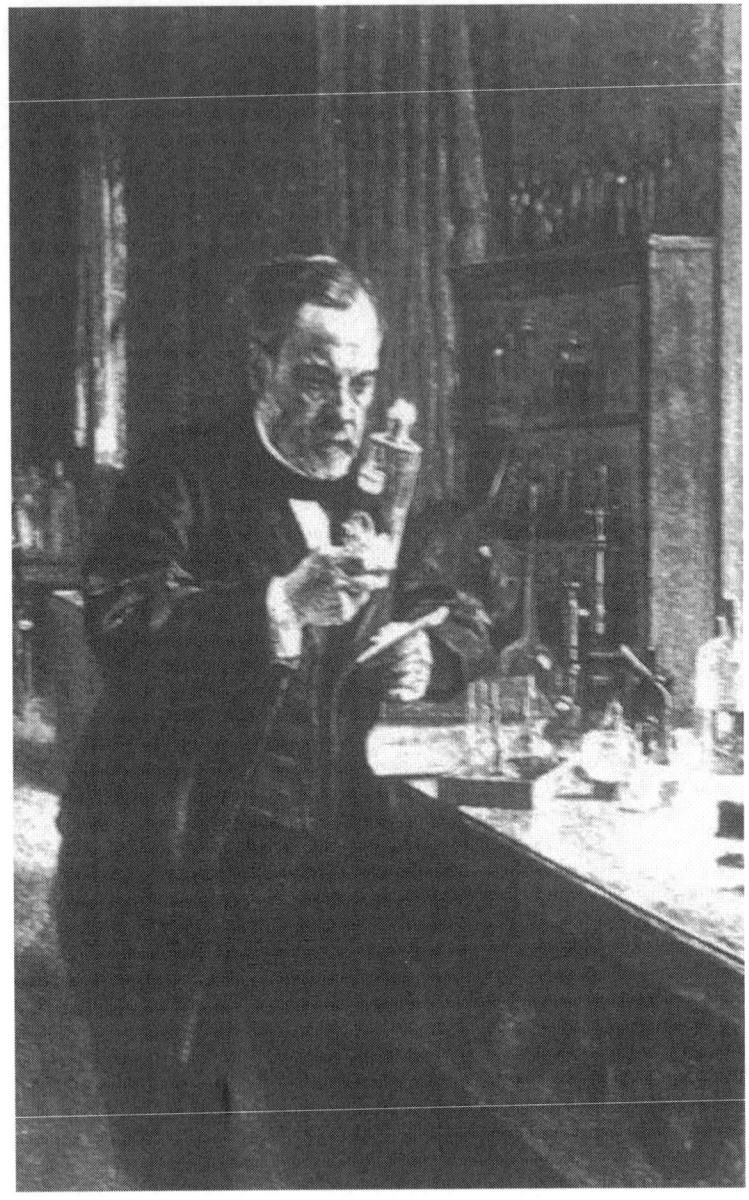

Louis Pasteur

Pasteur said, "Chance only favors the mind that is prepared."

Louis Pasteur (1822–1895)

Louis Pasteur had a humble upbringing. He was the son of a tanner who had fought in Napoleon's army. Young Louis Pasteur had some talent with drawing, but he wanted to become a teacher. In 1840 he received a degree and taught mathematics. In 1842 he obtained a science degree. Interestingly, his test scores in chemistry were considered mediocre. Nevertheless, in 1847 he achieved a doctor of science degree and later became a professor of physics in Dijon in 1948. He then was appointed professor of chemistry at Strasbourg, at Lille, for the greater part of twenty years

Louis Pasteur had no formal medical training and did not attend school for a medical degree, but his life's work aligned the laboratory with practical problem solving like no other scientist ever at the time. Along with Jenner's work on variolation (small pox vaccination), Pasteur's work helped lay the foundation for modern vaccinations. Pasteur also elucidated that microscopic bacteria were the etiology of many diseases.

His discoveries were many. In 1848, he did the first experiments in stereochemistry and crystallography with studies on tartaric acid. Then, when the wine and beer industries in France were distraught over "putrid spirits," he discovered the process of fermentation and bacterial putrefaction and solved the problem by teaching a new technique called pasteurization—heating to kill putrefactive factors. Pasteur unequivocally proved that germ theory was correct; this was controversial and many believed in spontaneous generation prior to Pateur's work.

In 1865 to 1868, he worked on silkworm disease, which was destroying the French silk industry. In three short years, he found there were two causative agents and found ways to prevent both. Subsequently, the silk industry was again able to prosper because of Pasteur's economy-saving work in this area.

In 1868, after his above scientific accomplishments, Pasteur had a stroke. He had a prolonged paralysis and recovery period, but when he returned to work he was considered more of a bacteriologist than a chemist and became one of the pioneers of immunology.

After recovering from his stroke, he isolated both the causative agent of anthrax (splenic fever in sheep and cows) and chicken cholera. Not only was he able to isolate both organisms, but he was able to produce a vaccine from a weakened form of both microbes.

Perhaps his most famous discovery came in 1885, when he developed a rabies vaccine from the spinal tissues of infected rabbits. On July 6, 1885, nine-year-old Joseph Meister was bitten fourteen times by a rabid dog. After fourteen injections, Pasteur's vaccine saved Joseph's life. Several months later, a young man named Jupilles fought off a rabid dog to protect several of his comrades. Again, Pasteur's vaccine saved the man's life. A statue of Jupilles fighting bravely against a rabid dog stands outside the Pasteur Institute in Paris.

In 1868, after the many successes of his rabies vaccine, the Pasteur Institute was built, where he worked for his remaining years. We have great gratitude for his pioneering work in the vaccination and prevention of infectious diseases. As a result of Pasteur's revolutionary work, we have developed vaccines based on his fundamental principle that a weakened form of an organism often incurs immunity but not infection, and when a person is exposed to the full, virulent form of a microbe after receiving a vaccination, illness does not ensue.

Further, Pasteur's monumental work on putrefaction was read by Joseph Lister, who put the pieces together to solve the puzzle of postsurgical infections, a common problem at the time. Lister was to discover and advocate antiseptic technique, which significantly reduced postsurgical infections and dramatically decreased deaths after surgies.

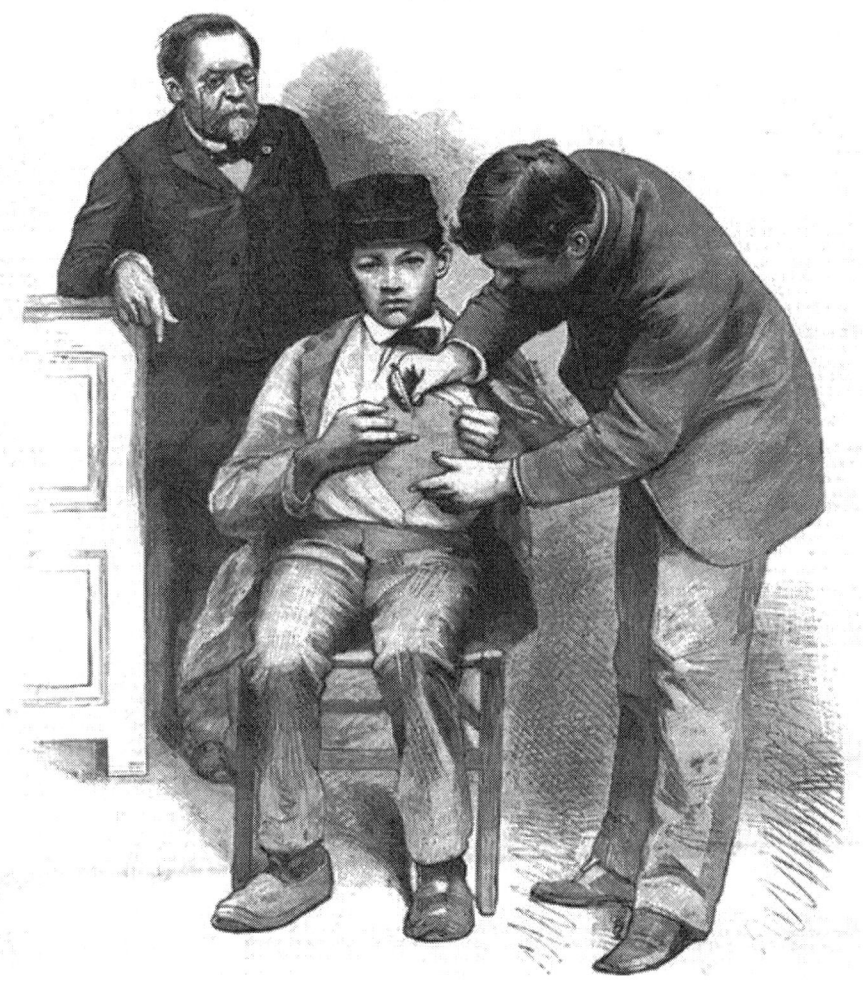

Boy receiving rabies vaccine as Pasteur observes

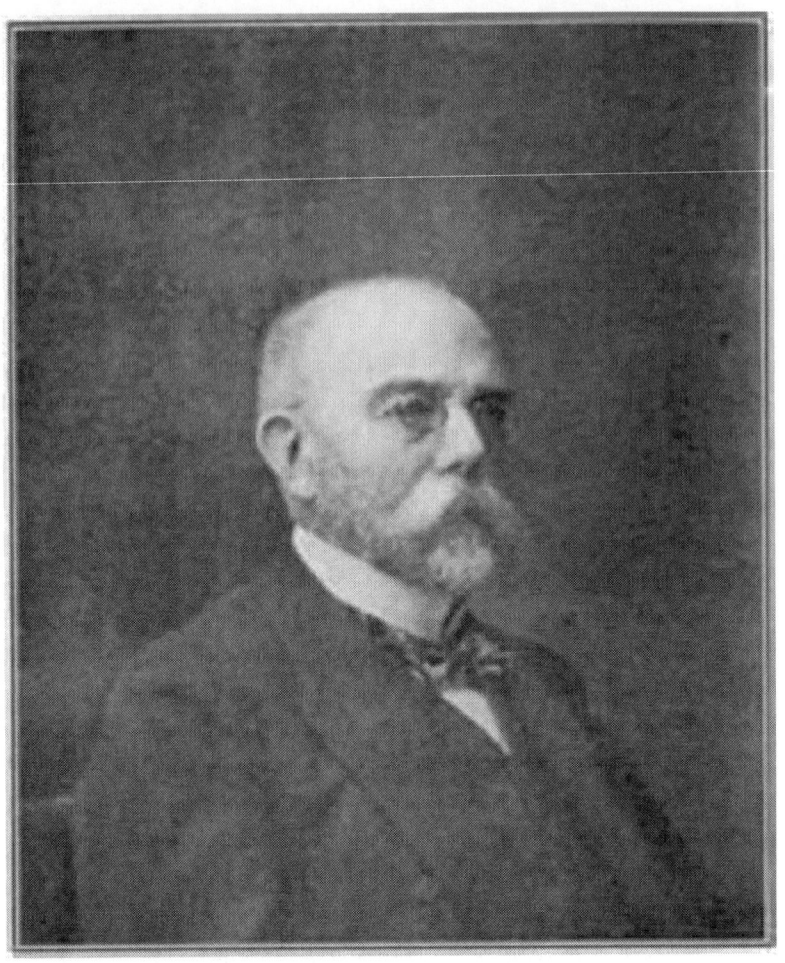

Robert Koch

Robert Koch (1843–1910)

Robert Koch was a practicing country physician who studied microorganisms in his spare time. He discovered the sporulation of anthrax. He unlocked the etiology of wound infections, cholera, Egyptian opthalmia, and sleeping sickness. He developed Koch's postulates for isolating bacteria and was the first to isolate tuberculosis.

Koch's postulates:

1. The microorganism must be found in all organisms suffering from the disease, but not in healthy organisms. (He later found that some people were asymptomatic carriers and the first postulate was not always true.)
2. The microorganism must be isolated from a diseased organism and grown in pure culture.
3. The cultured microorganism should cause disease when introduced into a healthy organism.
4. The microorganism must be reisolated from the inoculated, diseased experimental host and identified as being identical to the original specific causative agent.

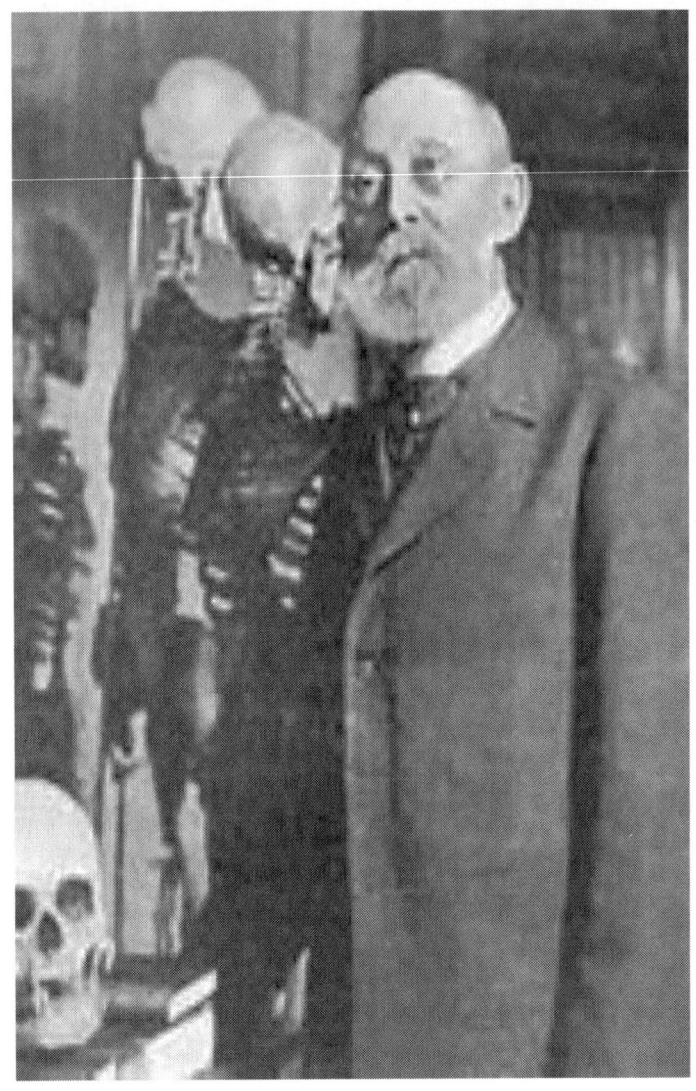

Rudolf Virchow

Rudolf Virchow (1821–1902)

Rudolf Virchow was the son of a prosperous farmer and graduated in 1843 from the University of Germany in Berlin. His efforts were concentrated in the study of pathology. In 1858 he wrote *Cellular Pathology*, which shocked the medical community because he claimed that disease arose from a cellular level, with damage to individual cells and not the entire organism. He revolutionized the diagnosis of disease, helping open new fields of bacteriology, immunology, and biochemistry. In 1856, he was given a full professorship at the Pathological Institute. He was also a political activist and a pioneering anthropologist, and he assisted his friend Heinrich Schielmann on excavations of the ancient city of Troy.

He studied blood and its clotting, including embolism. In addition, he studied nerves, muscles, and infectious diseases such as diphtheria, tuberculosis, leprosy, and typhus. One man remarked that Virchow, through his discoveries of pathology at the microscopic level, did more to advance medicine than anyone else before his time.

Today, medical students remember him for his discovery of the three risk factors—called Virchow's triad—that contribute to blood clots:

1. Venous stasis
2. Endothelial injury
3. Hypercoagulable states

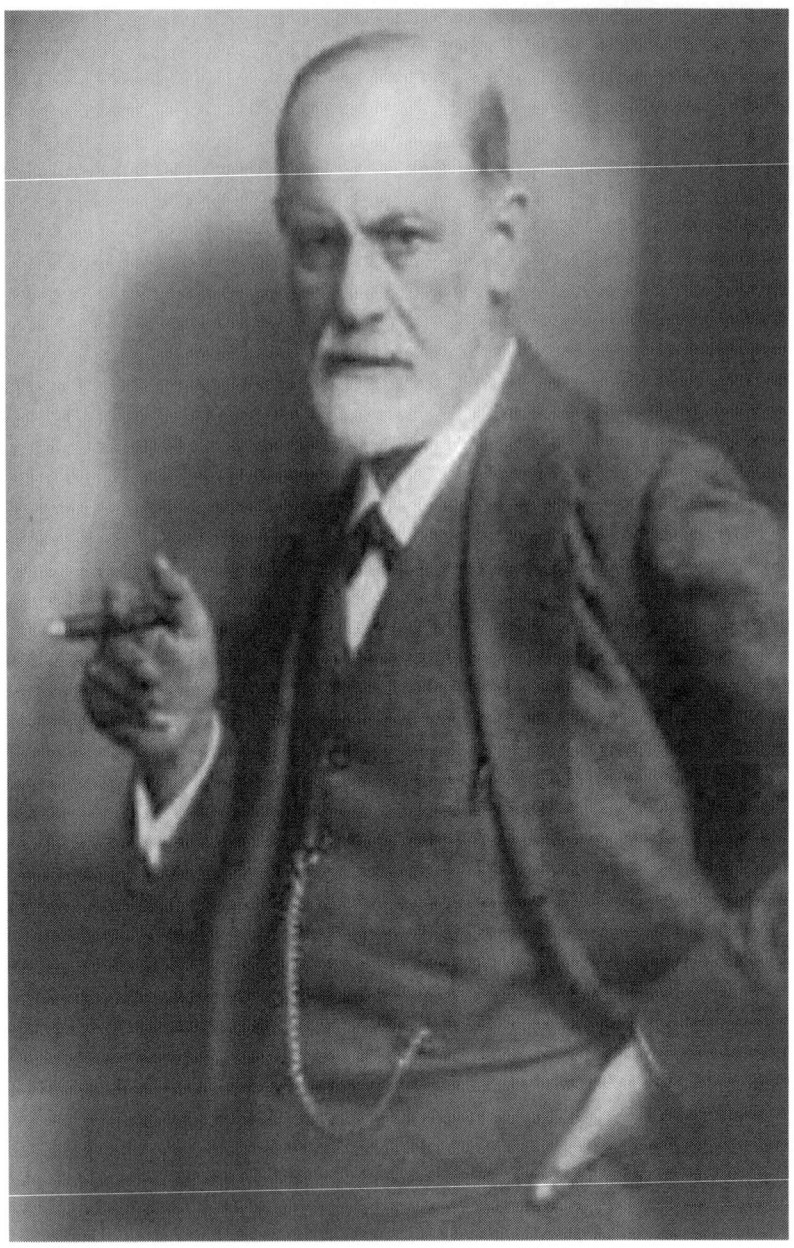

Sigmund Freud

Sigmund Freud (1856–1939)

The body does not function well when the mind is ill. Not until Sigmund Freud's controversial theories appeared, did the connection between the conscious and unconscious thoughts and their effects on the human body were linked. In Freud's own words, his work was to "agitate the sleep of mankind."

Born of Jewish descent, he lived near and attended the University of Vienna, where he obtained his medical degree in 1881. After specializing in neurology, he took an interest in hypnosis and developed theories of the unconscious mind and how repression played a role in the protection of the ego.

Freud was often an outcast in the medical community during his time, as were others like William Harvey, who threatened to change the teachings of Galen, and like Semmelweis for his views on handwashing to prevent sepsis. These doctors challenged tradition with new science and theories that were often met with resistance when first introduced.

Freud developed psychoanalysis, which brought a more humane approach to mental illness. Freud's work has helped us to better understand the many intricacies and complex circuits of the human mind. In addition, people began to understand the reasons for anxiety and how it could make them sick.

After a career of developing theories and concepts about how the human mind works, Freud was stricken with oral cancer in 1923. (He smoked cigars, sometimes a box a day.) . He had nearly 30 surgeries over the years for the cancer but continued to smoke cigars. Prior to the cancer he had written *Interpretation of Dreams*, *The Ego and the*

Id, and *Beyond the Pleasure Principle.* After 1923, he continued to work and make contributions to understanding the human mind. Some historians believe Freud was addicted to cocaine at one time. He stopped using it, and his reputation was tainted for some time until he stopped recommending it to patients for depression.

Freud's daily routine is said to have consisted of seeing patients from 8 am until noon, then he ate lunch at 1 o'clock Then he saw patients again from 3 in the afternoon until 9 at night. He also exercised going for a brisk walk daily. He had six children and his daughter Anna Freud became a well-known psychologist/psychiatrist as well.

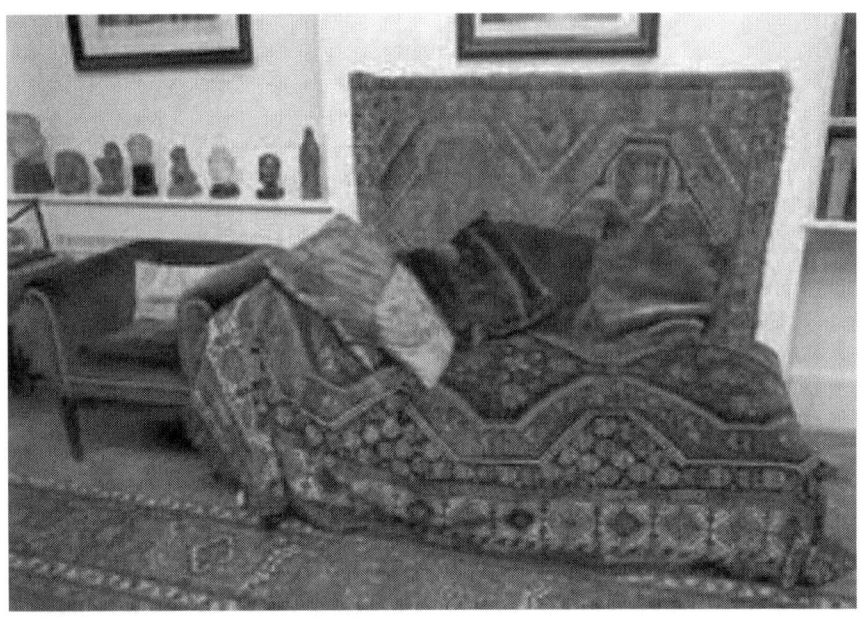

Sigmund Freud's couch for psychoanalysis.
Note the statues on the shelf. He collected
Greek and Roman artifacts.

As the German Nazis were nearing Vienna during World War II, Freud emigrated to Paris and then to London. He died in London on September 23, 1939 at the age of 83, after asking his physician to give him a lethal injection of morphine.

Sigmund Freud is often called the father of psychoanalysis, and shined a bright light on the newer branches of medicine: psychology and psychiatry.

Freud was a prolific writer and from 1891 to 1938 wrote and published over 120 books and articles. Here is a partial list of Sigmund Freud's writings, some of which are still available today:

1891 Aphasia
1895 Studies on Hysteria
1896 The Aetiology of Hysteria
1899 An Autobiographical Note
1900 Interpretation of Dreams
1904 The Psychopathology of Everyday Life
1905 Jokes and the their Relation to Unconscious
1905 Three essay on the Theory of Sexuality
1908 "Civilized" Sexual Morality and Modern Nervous Illness
1910 Leonardo da Vinci and a Memory of his Childhood
1912 Recommendations to Physicians Practicing Psycho-analysis
1912 The Dynamics of Transference
1913 Totem and Taboo: Resemblance Between the Psychic Lives of Savages and Neurotics
1914 On Narcissism
1914 On the History of the Psycho-Analytic Movement
1915 Repression
1915 The Unconscious
1917 Mourning and Melancholy
1920 Beyond the Pleasure Principle
1923 The Id and the Ego
1930 Civilization and it's Discontents
1938 Moses and Monotheism

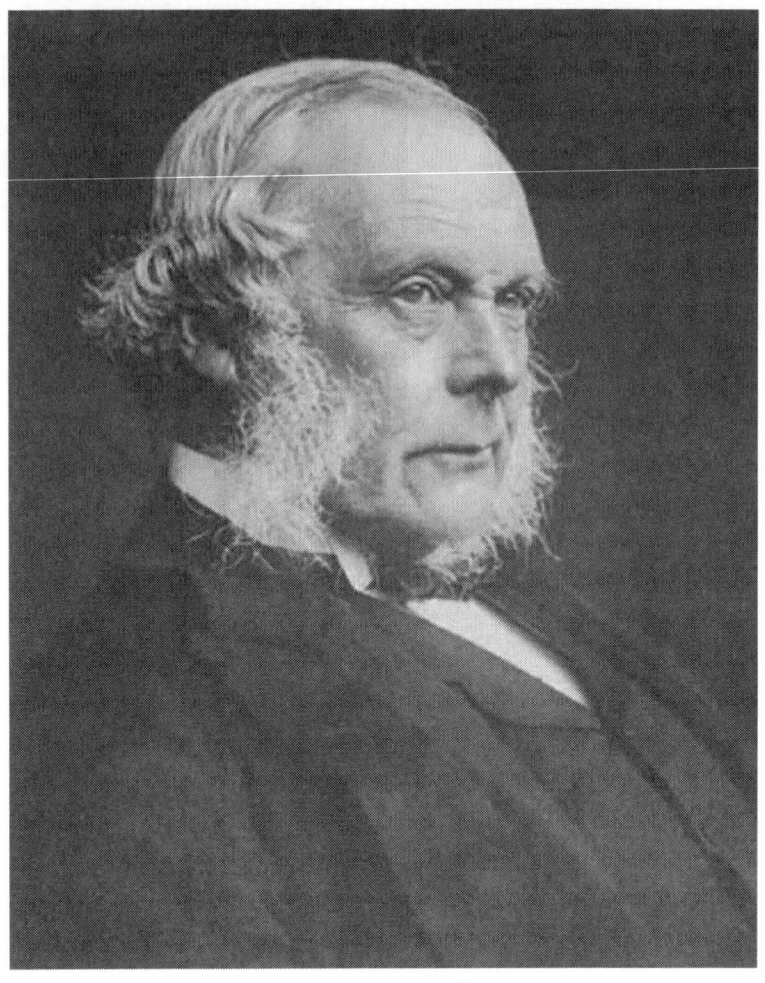

Joseph Lister

Joseph Lister (1827–1912)

Painless surgery using chloroform became more commonplace due to the efforts of two American dentists, William T. G. Morton and Horace Wells, and a contribution by an American surgeon, Crawford W. Long in 1846. The problem of putrefaction, the infection of postsurgical wounds, still took 40 to 50 percent of patients lives who underwent surgical procedures. When King George IV of England asked surgeon Astley Cooper to remove a cyst from the king's head, this successful surgeon was in fear for his career and livelihood because postoperative infections after many minor surgeries ended in the death of the patient. In the case of the cyst removal, perhaps because of the excellent blood supply of the scalp, no infection occurred, and Cooper was subsequently knighted for his daring operation. Such was the atmosphere of surgery in the nineteenth century.

Joseph Lister was an English physician and surgeon who, after reading the discovery on putrefaction of beer and wine by Pasteur, noted that it was caused by microbes and not a chemical reaction. He applied a similar theory to that of postsurgical wounds, but he took it one step further and postulated the possibility of wound infections being due to airborne microbes.

Lister observed that closed-bone fractures rarely led to infections, and open fractures in which the bone breaks through the skin usually became infected. In August 1865, his first experiment with carbolic acid was carried out. An eleven-year-old boy, James Grenless, presented to the Royal Infirmary in Glasgow with an open-tibia fracture after a carriage wheel ran over his leg. Lister used a lint bandage soaked in carbolic acid to cover the wound. The leg was splinted, and the open wound subsequently closed without developing an infection. Quite often a wound injury like this would have resulted in amputation. More open fractures were treated similarly, with successful results. Lister believed that perhaps he was onto something important.

With encouragement from his first studies, Lister applied his methods to psoas abscesses and then to amputations. In 1867 he published and introduced his landmark discovery of antisepsis. It was published in *Lancet* and entitled *The Antiseptic System: On a New Method of Treating Compound Fracture, Abscess, etc., with Observations on the Conditions of Suppuration.*

Lister's new rigid standard of *sterile technique* was followed during each operation he performed. He adhered to handwashing in a one-to-twenty dilution of carbolic acid prior to surgery. Further, he required that a continuous spray of carbolic acid mist cover the surgical field. He then placed gauze soaked in carbolic acid on incisions and wounds after surgery. This was all revolutionary.

As with most new surgical innovations, Lister's new methods were met with resistance by other surgeons. Theodore Billroth, a well-acclaimed surgeon who performed for large audiences in the surgical theater, doing surgery in his blood-stained coat at blazing speed and with bare hands, told his friend Volkman in 1874 that if Volkman wasn't so energetic to use anti-septic and sterile precautions, he would think the whole thing was a swindle. Yet the seed was planted, and as the newer generation of physicians were trained in Lister's antiseptic techniques, they too had fewer battles with postsurgical infections. Of course, today we routinely practice aseptic techniques to prevent surgical wound infections.

Joseph Lister's wife was his constant companion and a lifelong and excellent collaborator. Agnes Syme Lister was the daughter of his first mentor and was an indefatigable friend and assistant. In their house, they had their kitchen converted into a laboratory with test tubes and microscopes. In Lister's later years, his wife was his avid fly-fishing partner and bird-watching companion.

Before his death, Lister was well decorated, being the first doctor honored with the title of baron.

With chloroform, painless surgeries could be carried out. With Lister's aseptic techniques, surgeries were safer (although still with risk) than at any other time previous in the history of medicine. Joseph Lister is known as the father of antiseptic surgery.

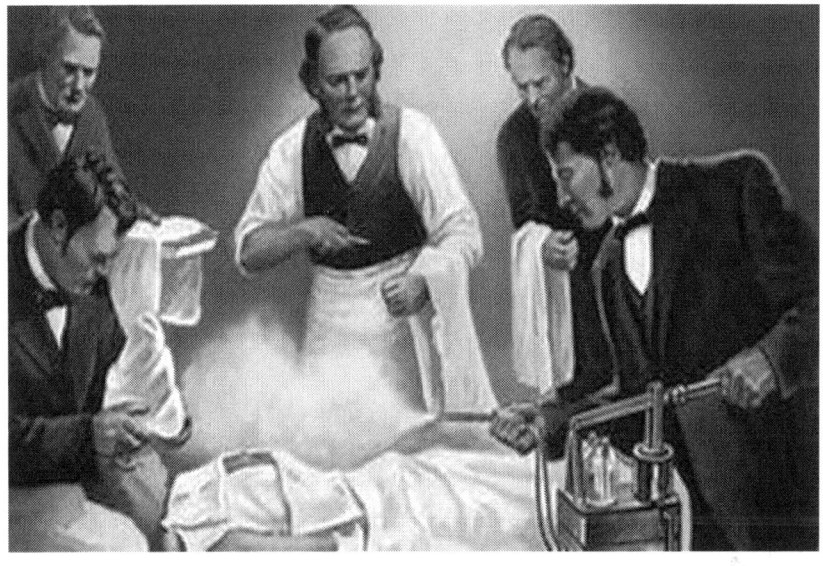

Joseph Lister having antiseptic sprayed onto his surgical field. A sterile operation meant less postoperative infections and less deaths from surgeries.

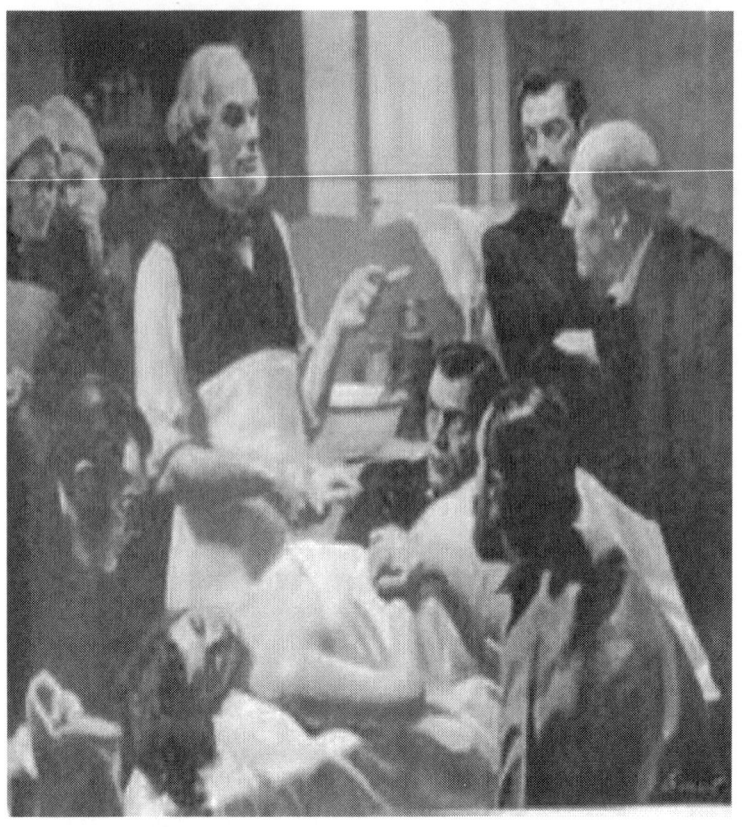

Joseph Lister performing surgery

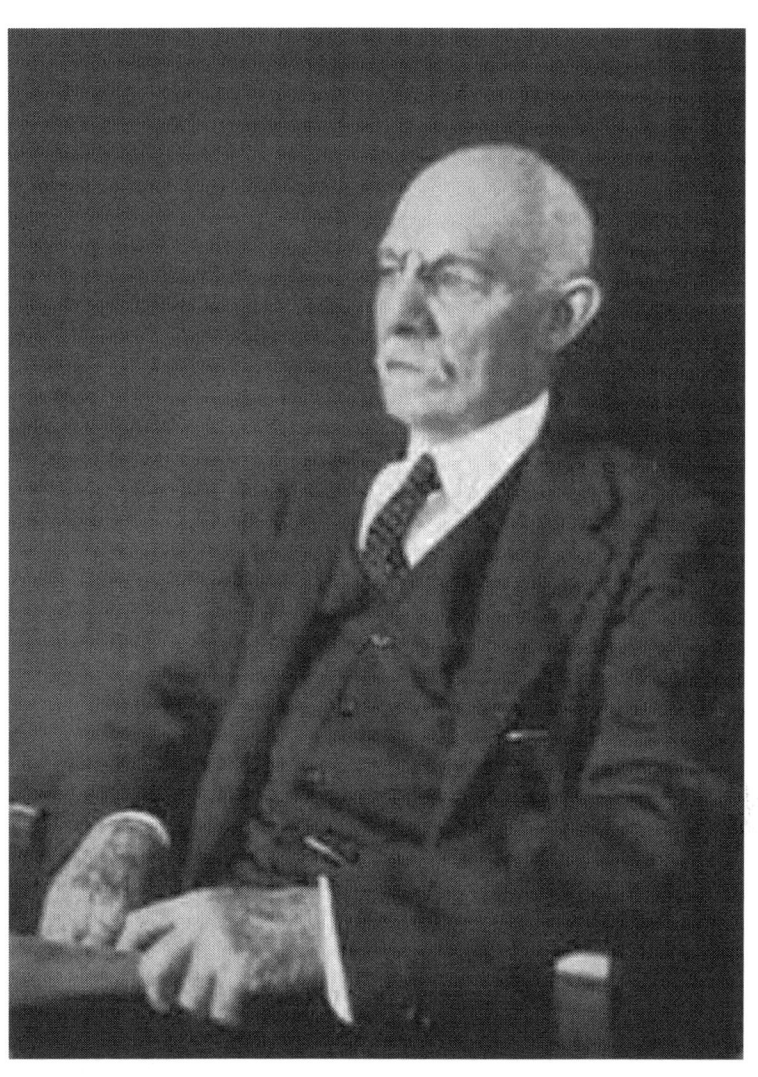

William Stewart Halsted

William Stewart Halsted (1852–1922)

William Halsted played for the Yale football team in 1874, played shortstop for the baseball team, and rowed on the crew team. He was the son of rich parents. He attended Yale for three years. Then he matriculated into medical school, spending three years at the College of Physicians in New York, in a class of 550 students. After his medical school training, he traveled to Vienna. While there, Halsted spent two years studying under Theodore Billroth, after which he returned to New York.

Returning to New York, Halsted quickly established himself as an excellent surgeon with high standards. At Bellevue Hospital in New York, he erected a tent adjacent to the hospital proper because Halsted wanted a facility in which he could ensure aseptic conditions.

Although a fine surgeon with a large and busy practice, he participated in anesthetic experiments that led to a lifelong addiction to narcotics, right up until his death.

In 1846, Dr. Karl Koller, at the suggestion of Sigmund Freud, did experiments proving the anesthetic qualities of cocaine when placed in solution. Halsted read of these and recruited colleagues and medical students for additional experiments. Perhaps unaware of the addictive qualities, many in the group became addicted, as did Halsted. A boating trip to "dry out" and two admissions to Butler Hospital—the latter for eight months—were not enough to rid him of the addiction. He subsequently became addicted to morphine, perhaps while in recovery from his cocaine addiction at Butler Hospital.

Halsted left New York in 1886 to work at the new Johns Hopkins University. He was thirty-six years old. He went to work in the laboratory under the watchful eye of the well-known pathologist William Welch. When the first surgical position opened, Halsted was given a temporary post as a surgeon. Halsted's skills were exceptional, and two years later he was named surgeon in chief and full professor.

He developed a rigorous course for training with a pyramid system at the new Johns Hopkins. Harvey Cushing was perhaps his most famous student, who helped develop the specialty of neurosurgery. Halsted graduated a "house surgeon" at the top of the pyramid, each after spending eight years on average in training with him. Among Halsted's contributions were his pioneering work with local anesthesia using cocaine, perfecting the repair of hernias, using metal clamps for occluding large vessels, and initiating the use of rubber gloves during surgery, which is now standard practice. He was also a proponent of blood transfusions and aseptic technique. His name still stands in surgical circles with the Halsted procedure, also known as a radical mastectomy.

Some site his Halsted principles, which are the basic principles of surgical technique regarding tissue handling. They include:

Gentle handling of tissue

Meticulous hemostasis

Preservation of blood supply

Strict aseptic technique

Minimum tension on tissues

Accurate tissue apposition

Obliteration of dead space

When Halsted was seventy years old, he needed surgery for gallbladder disease to remove a gallstone in one of his bile ducts. Two of his previous house surgeons left their practices to operate on their mentor. After the surgery, Halsted developed gastrointestinal bleeding and received a blood transfusion. He then developed pneumonia, which weakened him further. Several days later, he died, on September 7, 1922.

Halsted never was to overcome his addictions, first to cocaine and then to morphine. After being appointed the first surgeon at Johns Hopkins, Dr. William Osler wrote, "He had never been able to reduce the amount (of morphine) to less than three grains per day." Despite his personal affliction, William Halsted accomplished many great advances in surgery and truly deserves recognition as one of America's greatest surgeons.

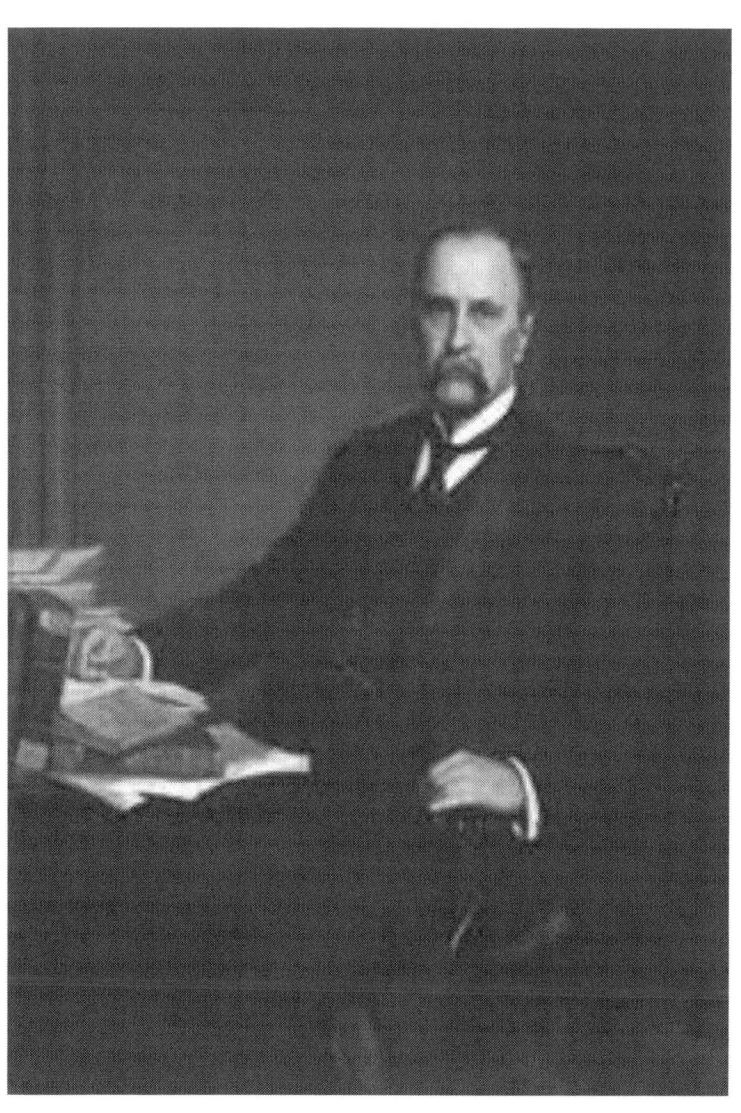

William Osler

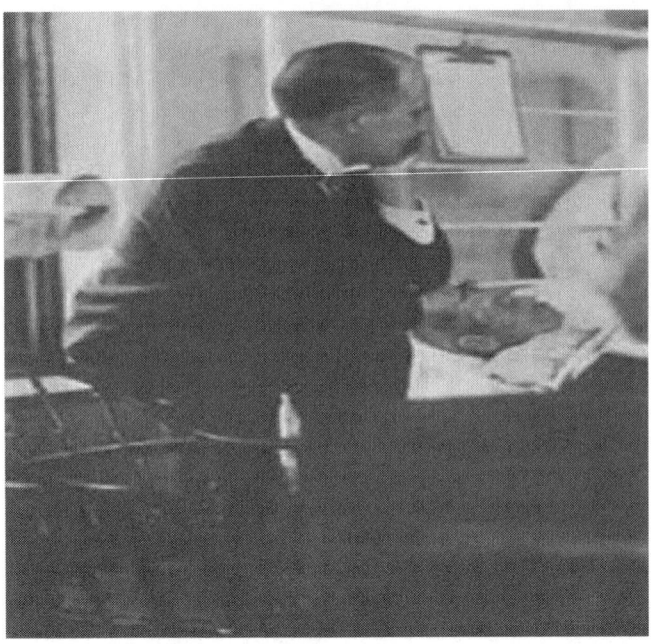

William Osler said, "Medicine should begin with the patient, continue with the patient, and end with the patient."

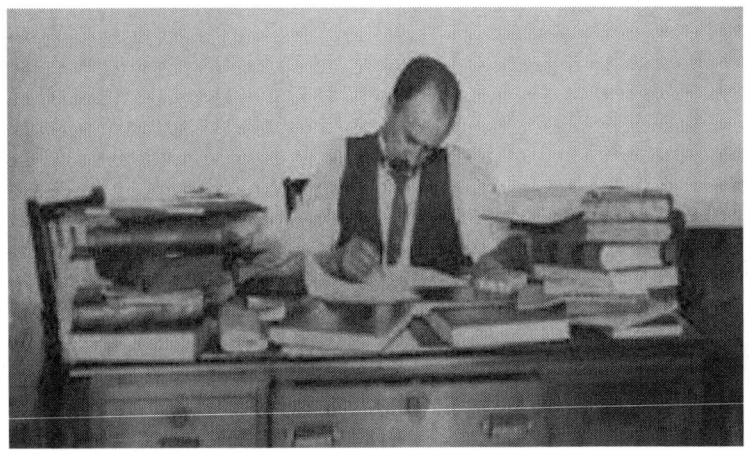

Osler writing at his desk

William Osler (1849–1919)

William Osler was the first professor of medicine at Johns Hopkins University. He trained at McGill in Montreal, and after going to Europe for further study, he returned to improve medical education and develop it into the university system and structure that it is today. For the first time, students were taken to the wards, and teaching rounds with an attending physician were conducted. The first class was admitted to Johns Hopkins in 1893.

While teaching and helping to develop criteria for acceptance to medical school, he wrote *Principles and Practice of Medicine*, which was the bible of medical education for over four decades. He also helped produce and edit the *Baltimore Circular*, which provided a means of suggestion to improve medical education. Of an original 148 medical students starting under the guidance of his medical training standards, only eighty-six medical schools remained for the end of their training. New standards of medical education were set using Osler's Johns Hopkins as the new rigorous gold standard.

Osler's work inspired the funding of the Rockefeller Institute of Medicine in 1897. Osler thought one should not stay too idle and that "Every five years one should return to the bench for research."

His biography was written by William Cushing, himself advancing the art and science of neurosurgery. Osler was a bibliophile, procuring a voluminous library, and he wrote and studied about the history of medicine. Above all, he laid the groundwork for the training and medical education system we have today.

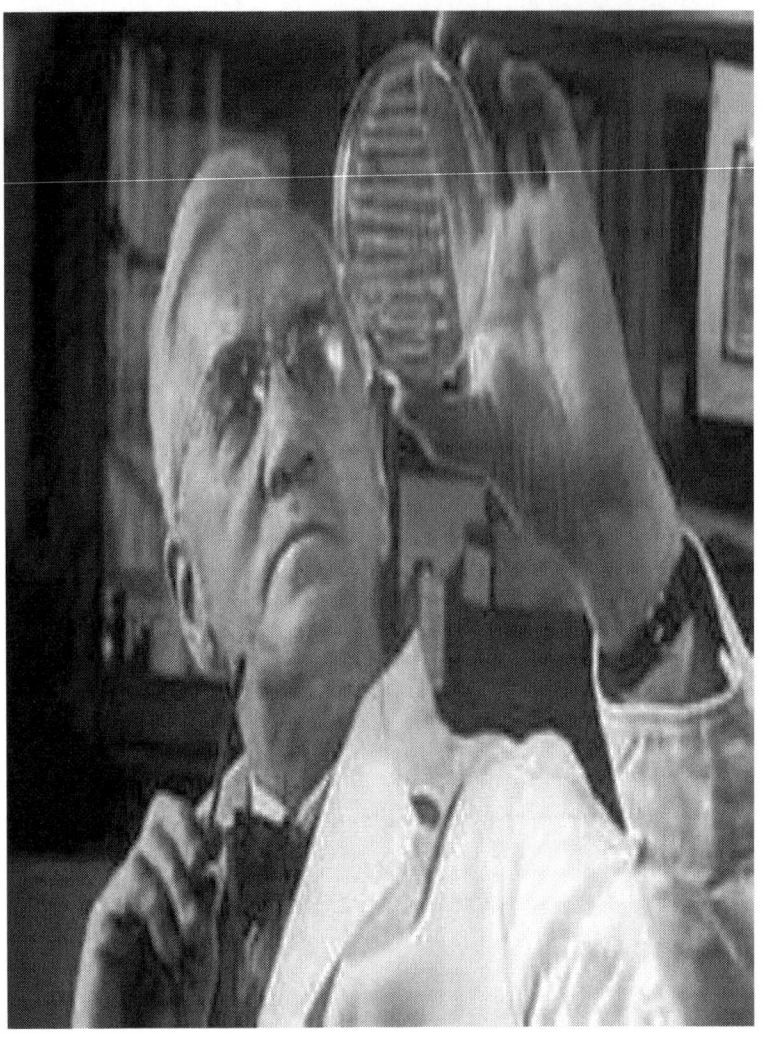

Alexander Fleming

Sir Alexander Fleming discovered penicillin.
Here he is examining a petri dish.

Sir Alexander Fleming (1881–1955)

Alexander Fleming was a Scottish biologist, pharmacologist, and botanist who discovered penicillin, beginning the modern era of antibiotics. His best-known discoveries were the enzyme lysozyme in 1923 and the antibiotic penicillin from the mold *Penicillium notatum*. For his work he shared the Nobel Prize in Physiology of Medicine with Howard Florey and Ernst Boris Chain.

In 1928, after going on vacation, Fleming returned to his laboratory and noticed that one culture was contaminated with a fungus and that the colonies of *Staphylococci* that had immediately surrounded it had been destroyed. He identified the mold, *Penicillium*, and deduced that it had released a substance that killed bacteria.

He investigated its antibacterial effect on many organisms and found it killed bacteria that caused strep throat, scarlet fever, pneumonia, meningitis, and diphtheria. Fleming published his discovery in 1929, in the *British Journal of Experimental Pathology*. It was immediately accepted as a significant contribution to science and medicine. The discovery of penicillin revolutionized medicine by making available the first laboratory-produced antibiotic.

Fleming also discovered very early that bacteria developed antibiotic resistance when too little penicillin was used or when it was used for too short a period. He cautioned about the use of penicillin in his many speeches around the world. He recommended not using penicillin unless there was a properly diagnosed reason. He recommended that if it were used, too little should never be used or for too short a period, since these are the circumstances in which bacterial resistance to antibiotics develops.

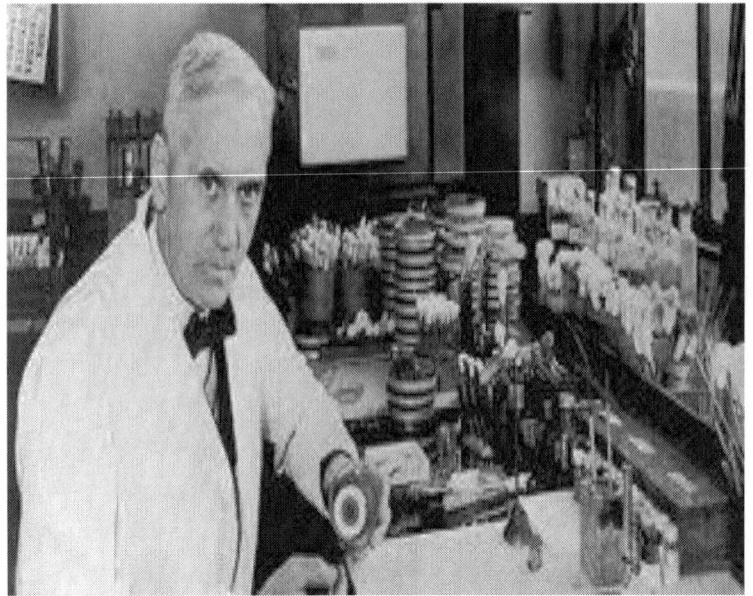

Sir Alexander Fleming in the lab

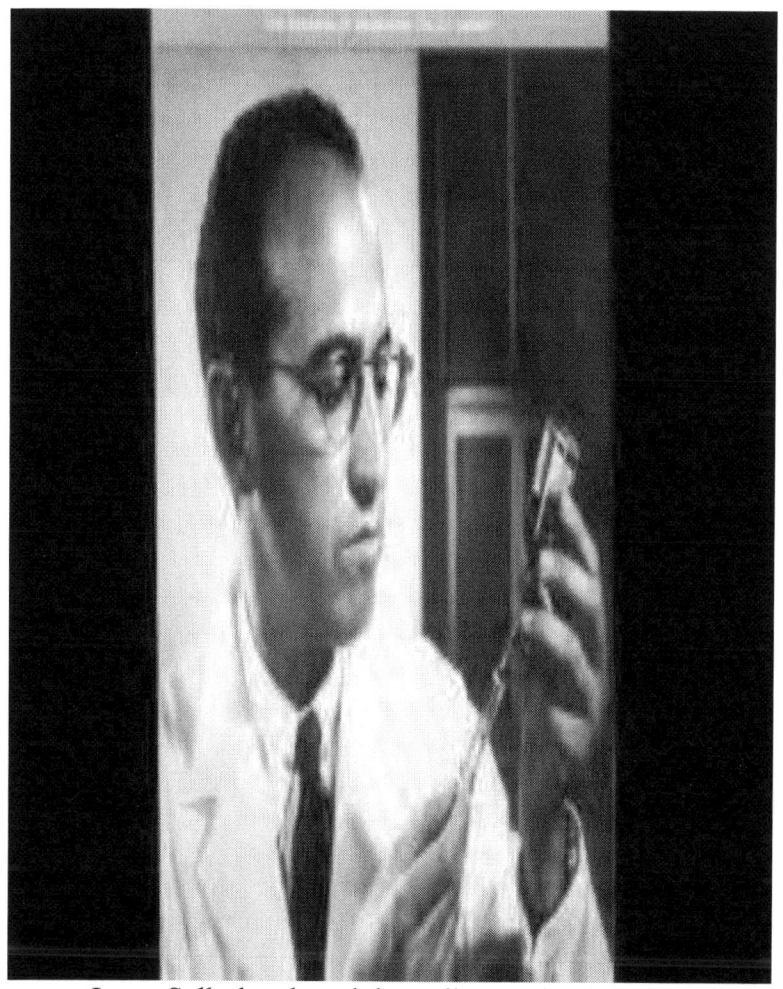

Jonas Salk developed the polio vaccine in 1955.

Jonas Edward Salk (1914–1995)

Jonas Salk developed the first successful polio vaccine and made it available to everyone in 1955. He was born in New York and attended New York University School of Medicine. Salk decided to enter into medical research instead of becoming a practicing physician.

After World War II, polio began causing illness and paralysis. Some suspected that even the president Franklin D. Roosevelt had polio. In 1952 an epidemic broke out that was the worst outbreak in the nation's history. Over three thousand people died, and more than twenty thousand were left with crippling paralysis. There were more than fifty thousand people afflicted with the virus in 1952 alone. Fear had spread that it was the beginning of a modern-day plague.

Salk began working at University of Pittsburgh School of Medicine in 1947. In 1948, he undertook a project funded by the National Foundation for Infantile Paralysis. Over the next seven years, he involved twenty thousand physicians and public health officers, sixty-four thousand school personnel, 220,000 volunteers, and over 1,800,000 schoolchildren to take part in clinical trials.

When the vaccine became available in 1955, he was asked who owned the patent to the vaccine, Salk replied, "There is no patent. Could you patent the sun?"

In 1960, he founded the Salk Institute for Biological Studies in La Jolla, California. He continued to conduct research and publish books, including *Man Unfolding* (1972), *The Survival of the Wisest* (1973), *World Population and Human Values: A New Reality* (1981), and *Anatomy of Reality: Merging of Intuition and Reason* (1983). In Salk's last years he sought to find a vaccine against HIV, the virus that causes AIDS.

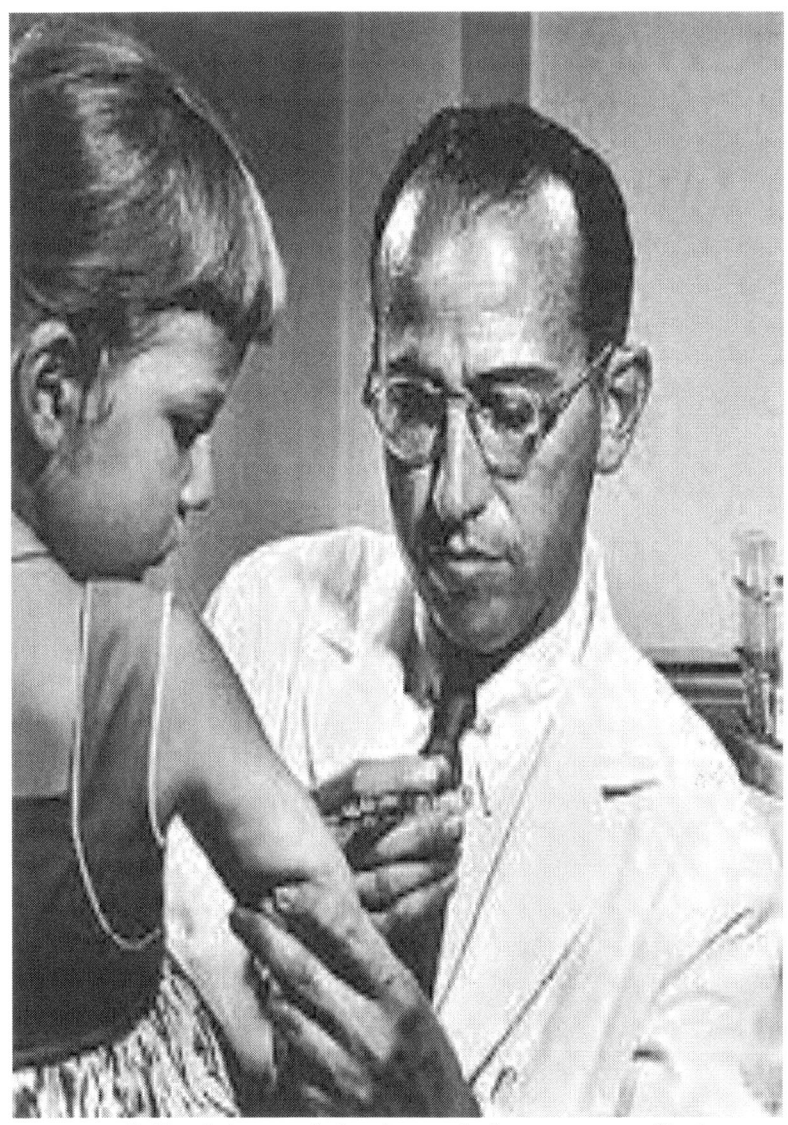

Salk giving an injection to help prevent polio

Understanding and learning about the history of medicine gives us a better appreciation and understanding of ourselves.

Partial List of References:

1. Great Medical Disasters – Dr. Richard Gordon
2. Call the Doctor: A Social History of Medical Men – E.S Turner
3. Devils, Drugs and Doctors – Haggard
4. The Alarming History of Medicine – Richard Gordon
5. Great Doctors – Henry G Sigerist
6. The Romance of Medicine – Logan Clendening
7. Louis Pasteur – Free Lance of Science
8. History of Medicine – Garrison 4th Ed
9. Bedside Manners – Edward Shorter
10. The Doctor – Truman
11. A History of Medicine – Jean Starobinski
12. A Pictoral History of Medicine – Otto Bettman

Famous Doctors

Famous Doctors

Printed in Dunstable, United Kingdom